Table of Contents

IV Training for EMTs

Section I

State Requirements for Colorado

Throughout your career in EMS, you will find that every state in the Union has its own requirements. Only Colorado requirements will be mentioned to give a frame of reference.

IV Class Purpose: Within the Practice Rules, it is stated that a *Colorado certified* Emergency Medical Technician (EMT), upon completion of an education program approved by the Colorado Department of Public Health and Environment (CDPHE) Emergency Medical and Trauma Services (EMTS) section and under the authorization (sponsorship) of a Colorado licensed physician, may establish a peripheral intravenous line, administer crystalloid fluids, collect venous blood samples, and administer certain medications. **Each student requires clinical experience before completing the EMT-IV/IO Therapy course.**

1. EDUCATION

a. Clinical experience shall consist of the following:
- no less than ten (10) successful venipunctures utilizing over-the-needle intravenous catheters
- No less than five (5) successful intraosseous placements on mannequins or live patients
- No less than five (5) successful intramuscular injections on mannequins or live patients

2. DURATION

a. Recommended 24 hours of classroom and practical training

3. Hands-on skills/Written testing

SKILLS PERMITTED UPON COMPLETION (WHEN INDICATED)

1. Human venipuncture for the following purposes:

- Determination of blood glucose measurements
- Collection of venous blood samples
- Initiation of intravenous therapy to include the following purposes
- Fluid replacement utilizing sterile crystalloid solutions
- Medication administration route utilizing sterile crystalloid solutions

2. Venous sites permitted shall be limited to peripheral veins (excluding external jugular) in both adults and children
3. Measurement and interpretation of blood glucose levels
4. Administration of intravenous dextrose
5. Administration of intravenous and atomized naloxone (Narcan)
6. Administration of nebulized albuterol (Proventil)

7. Administration of intravenous and oral dissolving tabs of ondansetron (Zofran)
8. Administration of intramuscular epinephrine 1:1,000
9. Intraosseous placement for the following purposes:
    - Fluid replacement utilizing crystalloid solutions for patients in extremis (cardiac arrest, etc.)
    - Medication administration

Expectations for EMT conduct and decorum encompass a wide range of behaviors, including but not limited to demonstrating compassion, empathy, and respect toward patients, colleagues, and the public. EMTs are also expected to maintain a demeanor that reflects the seriousness and sensitivity of their role, ensuring that their appearance, language, and actions contribute to a professional and therapeutic environment.

The scope and authority of Practice Rules for Emergency Medical Technicians (EMTs) are crucial to ensure that they provide care within the parameters of their training and legal boundaries. These rules dictate the permissible interventions and procedures EMTs can perform in the field. The regulatory bodies overseeing EMT practice in Colorado include the Colorado Department of Public Health and Environment (CDPHE) and state-level emergency medical and trauma services advisory councils. These bodies establish the certification requirements, scope of practice, and continuing education for EMTs.

Practice Rules shape EMTs' scope of service by setting clear guidelines on the level of care they can provide, which varies depending on their certification level (e.g., EMT-Basic, Advanced EMT, or Paramedic). These rules ensure patient safety, guide EMT education and influence the operational protocols of emergency medical services (EMS) organizations. Practice rules are determined by your governing Medical Director operating within any applicable Federal, State, or Municipal laws.

---

(1) EMTs are sponsored under a medical director after License/Certification verification, Credentialing within the agency, and understanding of Clinical Protocols and Standing Orders asserted by Field Trainers

(2) CDPHE regulations. Due to the medical nature of EMS, CDPHE's oversight of EMS medical directors is set forth in regulations promulgated by CDPHE's executive director (or by the chief medical officer if the executive director is not a physician).[60] These regulations define the duties and responsibilities of all EMS medical directors and the physician medical direction required for appropriate oversight of EMS providers.

(3) EMS medical directors must:

- Establish a continuous medical quality improvement (CQI) program for each EMS agency that is being supervised.
- Provide monitoring and supervision of the medical field performance of EMS providers.
- Ensure that all protocols issued by the medical director are appropriate for the certification or license and skill level of each EMS provider to whom the performance of medical acts is authorized and compliant with accepted standards of medical practice and
- Be familiar with the training, knowledge, and competence of EMS providers under his or her supervision and ensure that EMS providers are appropriately trained and demonstrate ongoing competency in all authorized medical acts.

In addition, a Colorado EMS medical director must be currently licensed in good standing to practice medicine in the state, be actively involved in the provision of EMS in the community served by the EMS agency being supervised, be actively engaged regularly with the EMS agency being supervised, and be trained in Advanced Cardiac Life Support, to list a few of the regulations.

The professionalism standards for EMTs, mainly when providing vascular therapy, are rooted in a combination of technical proficiency, ethical conduct, and interpersonal skills. These standards include maintaining current knowledge of best practices, upholding patient confidentiality, obtaining informed consent, and providing care with respect for each patient's dignity and autonomy.

Professionalism impacts patient care and public trust significantly. When EMTs adhere to professional standards, it enhances the quality and safety of patient care and fosters trust in the healthcare system. Public confidence in EMS is essential for effective community health services, and professional conduct by EMTs reinforces this trust.

Professionalism among EMTs is multifaceted, requiring medical and procedural knowledge and the capacity to manage emotional and cognitive demands, which are critical for maintaining public trust and delivering high-quality patient care.

Importance of Thorough Documentation in Patient Care Reports

- Clear identification of the patient and verification of the correct site and procedure to be performed.
- Detailed consent forms that outline the risks, benefits, and alternatives to the procedure.
- A pre-procedure checklist to ensure all necessary equipment and preparations are complete.
- Intraoperative notes that include a description of the procedure, any complications, and follow-up

Legal Implications of Accurate Record-Keeping

- Accurate documentation is legally required to demonstrate adherence to standards of care and informed consent.
- It provides a legal record that can protect healthcare providers in the event of malpractice claims.
- Incomplete or inaccurate records can lead to legal consequences, including fines and litigation.

Documentation Requirements for Invasive Procedures:

Indications, catheter size, location, successful or unsuccessful, **ESO narrative, and flowchart.**

Emergency Medical Technicians must be conversant with various legal terms that pertain to their duties and the broader healthcare context.

1. **Duty to Act**: The legal obligation of EMTs to provide care in certain situations, typically when on duty or if they are the first to arrive at the scene of an emergency.
2. **Standard of Care:** The level of care and judgment exercised by a reasonably prudent EMT under similar circumstances.
3. **Negligence**: A failure to act or act in a way that deviates from the standard of care, which causes harm to the patient.
4. **Informed Consent**: The legal process of obtaining permission from a patient before conducting a healthcare intervention after the patient has been informed of the risks, benefits, and alternatives.
5. **Implied Consent**: A legal concept where consent is inferred based on the situation, such as when a patient is unconscious and immediate medical intervention is necessary to preserve life or prevent further harm.
6. **Refusal of Care**: The right of a competent adult to refuse medical treatment, even if it may result in harm or death. (Refer to APEX form)
7. **Abandonment**: The unlawful termination of the EMT-patient relationship without ensuring the patient has been transferred to equal or higher medical authority.
8. **Confidentiality**: The requirement to keep patient information private and disclose it only with consent or when legally mandated.
9. **Advanced Directives**: Legal documents that outline a patient's preferences regarding medical treatment should they become unable to make decisions for themselves.

10. **Do Not Resuscitate (DNR)**: A legal order to not perform CPR or advanced cardiac life support if a patient stops breathing or their heart stops beating.
11. **Liability**: Legal responsibility for one's actions or omissions, which, in the case of EMTs, can pertain to patient care.
12. **Assault and Battery**: Performing a procedure without consent, which could be construed as assault or offensively touching the patient, is considered battery.
13. **Good Samaritan Laws**: Laws designed to protect healthcare professionals and ordinary citizens from liability when they provide care in good faith during emergencies.
14. **Scope of Practice**: The procedures, actions, and processes that a healthcare practitioner is permitted to undertake in keeping with the terms of their professional license.

Check on Learning

A new EMT pulled over at the scene of an accident and performed an emergency cric on a patient to restore their airway. Is this covered under the Good Samaritan Law?

True or False?

Good Samaritan Laws are designed to provide legal protection to bystanders who assist victims during emergencies, offering some level of immunity against civil damages if they act voluntarily, without expectation of remuneration, act in good faith, and within the scope of their training. An EMT acting outside of their scope will likely face disciplinary and legal action.

Ethical considerations in patient advocacy and care decisions are multifaceted, involving the protection of vulnerable patients, respect for autonomy, appropriate medical care, avoiding discrimination, and managing potential conflicts of interest. These considerations aim to balance procedural safeguards with the ethical imperatives of practice.

Protecting Vulnerable Patients: Ethical advocacy requires health professionals to safeguard the interests of those who cannot advocate for themselves due to age, illness, or social circumstances. This involves supporting patients' rights, wishes, and values and may require nurses to develop strategies to regain the courage to engage in advocacy, especially in end-of-life care situations [(Luca, Cavicchioli, & Bianchi, 2021)

Respect for Persons: Ensuring patients' autonomy and decision-making capabilities are respected is crucial. This involves informed consent discussions that not only address the medical aspects of care but also consider the patients' social, cultural, and personal values (Bjorklund & Lund, 2019)

Appropriate Medical Care: Ethical advocacy in nursing practice includes the provision of empathetic, responsible, and assertive communication to ensure patients receive appropriate and just medical care. This can involve challenging institutional norms and advocating for systemic change to improve the overall quality of healthcare (Heck, Carrara, & Mendes, 2022)

Safeguarding Against Discrimination: Advocates work to identify and correct inequalities in the delivery of health services, which is particularly important for marginalized or underserved populations. This includes promoting ethical considerations in nursing care to ensure decisions are made without discrimination and uphold patient rights, values, and confidentiality (Scott & Scott, 2020)

Managing Conflicts of Interest: Healthcare professionals need to recognize and manage any competing obligations or conflicting interests that may arise, particularly during a health crisis such as a pandemic. This involves prioritizing patient care while conserving resources and minimizing risks to healthcare workers and other patients (Bernstein, 2020)]

In practice, these ethical considerations translate into actions that range from direct patient care to broader policy advocacy, each aiming to uphold the dignity and rights of patients within the healthcare system. Healthcare professionals must navigate these ethical landscapes thoughtfully, balancing the needs of the individual with those of the community, particularly in challenging situations such as the COVID-19 pandemic (Moore et al., 2022)

Protocols and **standing orders** are guidelines for medical practices but serve different functions in emergency medical care.

Protocols are comprehensive guidelines that outline the process for assessment, treatment, and management of different medical conditions. These are often based on best practices and evidence-based medicine to guide Emergency Medical Technicians (EMTs) in delivering care.

Standing orders, on the other hand, are specific instructions authorized by a medical director that allow EMTs to administer treatments or medications without direct physician oversight at the moment of care. They are designed to expedite care, especially in critical situations where immediate action is needed and physician consultation is not feasible.

For EMT actions in the field:

Protocols direct EMTs by providing detailed guidance on evaluating patients and determining the necessary steps for treatment. They are like a roadmap for EMTs to follow in various medical situations.

Standing orders empower EMTs to take immediate actions based on their assessment and the patient's condition. They allow for quick intervention, which can be crucial in emergencies.
Examples of scenarios:

Protocol Scenario: An EMT follows a stroke protocol, which includes assessing the patient's symptoms, taking vitals, and following specific steps to ensure the patient is transported rapidly to a stroke center.

Standing Order Scenario: An EMT encounters a patient with a severe allergic reaction and, per the standing orders, administers epinephrine without waiting for direct physician approval, as the standing orders pre-authorize this action under such conditions.

Standing orders in emergency departments can significantly reduce disposition time by expediting medical decision-making (Hwang et al., 2016)

The use of standing orders by triage nurses can decrease patient length of stay and improve the efficiency of care in emergency settings (Samiedaluie et al., 2020)

Emergency medical services use standing order protocols to enable more efficient and accurate on-scene management by paramedics, although the need for online medical direction persists for complex decision-making (Rai et al., 2020)

To be compliant with regulations, EMT-IVs may initiate venipuncture for the following purposes:

Fluid Administration

Medication Administration
Lab draws for receiving facility

BSI

Emergency medical services (EMS) responders are a critical part of the nation's emergency response system and the front line of medical response. They provide medical treatment at the scene of an incident and are often among the first responders to arrive. As a result, EMS responders are also likely to be present on the scene before hazards are fully controlled and situational awareness is complete. Incident sites routinely contain evolving dangers that can harm emergency responders. (OSHA Best Practices Handbook, 2009)

OSHA published standards on EMS best practices and first responder awareness training. **Infection control** is an integral part of this. CDPHE publishes guidance on local public health threats, and agencies should do their best to stay aware of alerts regarding infectious diseases, their prevalence, and recognition.

OSHA also provides best practices for training and equipping EMS responders during the treatment and transport of potentially contaminated victims during HAZMAT or chemical/biological events.

"A final section addresses hazardous substance decontamination. Although EMS responders might not be assigned to a community's decontamination team, they should understand the process if they are to recognize ineffective decontamination procedures that could result in improperly decontaminating- ed patients – patients that EMS responders could be expected to treat and transport. Furthermore, OSHA believes that during a mass casualty incident, EMS responders could be assigned to assist with decontamination and would need to know how to perform effective patient decontamination." (OSHA, 2009)

This is specialized training that not many agencies engage in; however, for your awareness, it exists, and during your career, you might be called to participate in it.

Contact with blood or body fluids through broken skin is a standard transmission mode for blood-borne pathogens, including viruses like HIV and hepatitis B and C.

Inhalation of airborne pathogens: Diseases such as tuberculosis, influenza, and COVID-19 can spread through the air, particularly in enclosed spaces.

Direct skin or mucous membrane contact: Certain infections, like herpes simplex virus or conjunctivitis, can be spread through direct contact with the skin or mucous membranes. Understanding these transmission routes is crucial for implementing appropriate infection control measures and developing public health policies to prevent the spread of infectious diseases. (www.CDC.gov, 2024)

- **Transmission through contact with blood or body fluids**: Infectious diseases can be transmitted via contact with blood or body fluids through broken skin. To mitigate this risk, it is crucial to employ standard infection control practices, especially in healthcare settings (Jacob & Cummins, 2019).

- **Airborne transmission**: Pathogens can be transmitted by inhalation of small respiratory droplets, which can remain airborne for extended periods, emphasizing the importance of ventilation, air filtration, and mask-wearing to reduce this type of transmission (Drossinos & Stilianakis, 2020) (Morawska et al., 2020).

- **Direct skin or mucous membrane contact**: Direct contact with mucous membranes is a significant mode of transmission for pathogens, highlighting the need for protective measures such as gloves and face shields in situations with high risk of splash or spray of body fluids (Checchi et al., 2020).

Body Substance Isolation (BSI) practices in Emergency Medical Services (EMS) are paramount for several reasons:

- **Prevention of Nosocomial Infections**: BSI practices are essential for preventing nosocomial infections, as they involve barrier precautions, such as gloving when contact with potentially infectious bodily secretions is anticipated. This is critical in EMS settings where patients may have various infections (Lynch et al., 1987).
- **Protection of Healthcare Workers**: BSI practices protect healthcare workers from bloodborne pathogens such as hepatitis B and HIV, as well as other infectious agents. This is particularly important in EMS due to the high-risk nature of emergency interventions (Lynch et al., 1990).
- **Consistent Application of Precautions**: The BSI system is used for all patients, not just in response to specific diagnoses, promoting consistent application of precautions and reducing the risk of cross-contamination (Jackson & Lynch, 1991)

Safety culture in emergency medical services (EMS) involves organizational policies and procedures, individual professionalism, and teamwork.

Evidence:

- Prehospital nursing students' experiences indicate that patient safety events in EMS are often related to communication, verification, and teamwork, and such events are seldom reported in healthcare systems or patient files (Venesoja et al., 2022).

- Tools like the Emergency Medical Service Safety Attitude Questionnaire are highlighted for assessing patient safety culture in emergency settings, emphasizing teamwork, management support, and continuous improvement (Torrente & Barbosa, 2021).

- A survey based on the Agency for Healthcare Research and Quality's Surveys on Patient Safety Culture (SOPS) shows adequate psychometric properties to evaluate safety culture in EMS. It correlates with safety outcomes (Crowe et al., 2018).

- The lack of data collection on patient and provider safety in EMS indicates a need for better data collection and reporting to patient safety organizations (Leggio et al., 2016).

- Repeated surveys with the Emergency Medical Services Safety Attitudes Questionnaire can measure changes in safety climate over time, reflecting the impact of training and operational culture.

- Effective risk management and adherence to OSHA standards have significantly reduced work-related injuries (Neitzel, 2011).

- Training programs based on error reduction models have improved workplace safety and reduced occupational injuries (Koshy, Preustti, & Rosen, 2019).

- The establishment of OSHA has significantly decreased work-related deaths and illnesses, but continuous updates and resources are necessary for further reductions (Michaels & Barab, 2020).

- Studies have shown that OSHA inspections and penalties significantly reduce injury claims, suggesting the effectiveness of enforcement in improving workplace safety (Michaels, 2012).

Post-exposure prophylaxis (PEP) policies for Emergency Medical Services (EMS) personnel are essential in Colorado and elsewhere to prevent transmitting infectious diseases after potential exposure incidents.

Evidence:

- PEP is a crucial emergency treatment started after exposure to a pathogen, like blood or body fluid, to prevent infection, with guidelines suggesting initiation within 72 hours following potential exposure to diseases like HIV (Mahiba, 2021).

- A study discussed the risks of acquiring blood-borne viruses, indicating that the actual risk is lower than perceived, and highlighted the availability of effective PEP for diseases like Hepatitis B and HIV (Speers, 2014).

- Research on healthcare workers exposed to Middle East Respiratory Syndrome (MERS-CoV) suggests that PEP can reduce the risk of infection and is safe for use (Park, Lee, Son, Ko, Peck, & Jung, 2018).

- In Colorado, a study on PrEP and PEP application to populations at risk, including EMS personnel, aids in public health strategic planning for HIV prevention at state and county levels (Donnelly, Deem, Duffy, Watkins, Al-Tayyib, Shodell, Thrun, & Rowan, 2019).

Refrain from filling SHARPS containers. “**Filling above the fill line or more than ¾ full of the alternative container can increase the risk of a needlestick injury and a bloodborne pathogen exposure.**” (www.cdc.gov, 2024)

Section II
Anatomy and Physiology

Homeostasis is a fundamental concept in medicine, referring to the complex balance and constancy of all aspects of body function, including the coordinated regulation of fluids and cells to maintain a stable internal environment. This stability is essential for health. It is achieved through various mechanisms, including physiological regulation and response to environmental changes.

1. Origin and Definition: Homeostasis originates from the Greek words for 'same' and 'steady,' emphasizing its role in maintaining a stable internal environment despite external perturbations (Kontopoulou & Marketos, 2002)

2. **Physiological Regulation**: Modern interpretations of homeostasis go beyond its original formulation, incorporating the concept of allostasis, which describes the body's ability to

achieve stability through change, particularly in response to stress or threats to stability (Ramsay & Woods, 2014)

3. **Neural and Synaptic Control:** Homeostatic signaling in the nervous system, through modulation of synaptic efficacy and membrane excitability, plays a crucial role in constraining neural plasticity and maintaining neural function stability over time (Davis, 2006)

4. **Adaptive Homeostasis:** The concept of adaptive homeostasis describes the body's ability to temporarily adjust its homeostatic range in response to environmental stimuli, such as exercise or exposure to chemicals, thereby adapting to short-term changes while maintaining overall stability (Davies, 2016)

5. **Physiological Monitoring:** A time-series analysis of physiological monitoring data, like heart rate and blood pressure, can reflect homeostatic regulatory processes and help differentiate between regulated variables and physiological responses, providing insights into health and disease states (Fossion, Rivera, & Estañol, 2018)

6. **Homeostasis in Disease:** Disruptions in homeostasis lead to disease, and understanding the self-regulating processes of homeostasis is crucial for comprehending body function in both health and disease (Billman, 2013)

Homeostasis is a dynamic and complex process essential for maintaining a stable internal environment in the body. It involves various regulatory mechanisms, adaptations, and feedback loops that constantly adjust to keep the body in harmony.

Intracellular fluid: This is the fluid located within the cells.

Extracellular fluid: This fluid is outside the cells and includes **interstitial fluid**, which is between cells, and intravascular fluid, which is within the blood vessels.

The balance between these fluids is vital for cell function.

Maintaining the balance between intracellular and extracellular fluids is crucial for various physiological processes, including transporting nutrients, removing waste, and maintaining proper function and communication between cells.

____

____

____

____

____

____

____

Tonicity and **Osmolarity**

Osmolarity measures the total concentration of solute particles per liter of solution. It's a way to describe the solution's ability to draw water across a semipermeable membrane. Osmolarity considers all particles that contribute to a solution's concentration, including ions, sugars, and proteins. It's measured in osmoles per liter (Osm/L) or milliosmoles per liter (mOsm/L).

Tonicity describes how a solution affects the volume of cells by osmosis, considering only the solutes that cannot cross the cell membrane. It's a relative term comparing the solution outside the cell to the fluid inside it.

HYPERTONIC solutions cause the cell to shrink due to water shifting from INTRAcellular to EXTRAcelluar.

ISOTONIC solutions are balanced. Water is equal on both sides of the cellular membrane.

HYPOTONIC solutions cause the cell to bloat and even lyse due to fluid shifting from EXTRAcellular to INTRAcellular.

- ISOtonic solutions are the same tonicity as human blood
    - NS, LR
- HYPOtonic solutions have a lower electrolyte concentration than blood
    - 0.45%NS
    - Force fluid into the cells
- HYPERtonic solutions have higher concentrations of electrolytes than blood
    - 3% NS
    - Pull fluid from cells into circulating volume

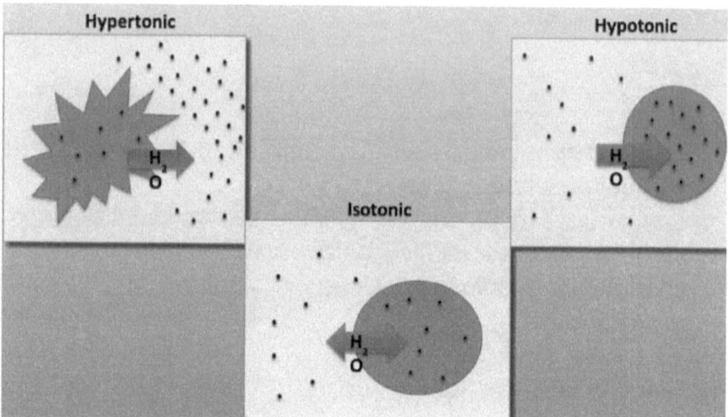

Isotonic: Same osmolarity as body fluids.

Hypotonic: Lower osmolarity than body fluids.

Hypertonic: Higher osmolarity than body fluids.

Summarized,

Isotonic solutions cause no net water movement into or out of cells, maintaining cell volume.

Hypotonic solutions lead to water moving into the cells, causing them to swell, which can be useful in treating dehydration but risky if it leads to cell lysis (bursting).

Hypertonic solutions lead to water moving out of the cells, causing them to shrink, which can be used to reduce cell swelling or edema but can be dangerous if it causes excessive cell dehydration.

Fluid Therapy Solutions

The choice of resuscitation fluid, whether crystalloid or colloid, significantly impacts the distribution of fluids in the body and can affect patient outcomes.

Crystalloids distribute in the extracellular space and are preferred for treating dehydration or maintaining fluid balance. Their low cost and ease of use make them a common choice, but they may increase edema (M. Saraghi, 2015)

Crystalloid solutions

- Isotonic: Same tonicity as human blood
- Examples: Normal saline, Lactated Ringer's
- Hypotonic: Lower concentrations of electrolytes than blood
- Fluid shifts from vascular to interstitial space
- Hypertonic: Higher concentrations of electrolytes than blood
- Fluid shifts into the vascular space

Colloids maintain circulatory volume due to larger molecules that remain in the intravascular space longer. However, they may cause adverse reactions and are not necessarily superior in expanding plasma volume in critically ill patients ([J. Vincent, 2019)

Colloid solutions

- **Albumin**
- Colloid solution derived from human blood donations
- used for hypovolemia, burns, surgical procedures
- **Hetastarch**
- Synthetic colloid solution
- Hespan (6% hetastarch in saline)
- Synthetic colloid made from corn
- Expansion equivalent to Dextran or Albumin
- Lower risk of allergic reaction than Dextran
- Hextend (6% hetastarch in Lactated Ringers)

- Effective for plasma expansion
- Incompatible with sodium bicarb and calcium products (blood)
- Do not give to pediatric patients
- **Dextran**
- Used when blood is unavailable
- Fluid Choice: The choice of fluid can affect fluid responsiveness and has been associated with differences in postoperative complications and the need for renal replacement therapy ([A. Joosten et al., 2018)

- Safety Profile: Colloids, mainly hydroxyethyl starch, have been linked to an increased risk of acute kidney injury and coagulopathies, challenging their use in fluid resuscitation (Dava Cazzolli & J. Prittie, 2015). Some older literature on trauma resuscitation might reference them, but they are not in common practice anymore.

While colloids may offer more immediate volume expansion, crystalloids are generally safer and preferable for most situations, particularly critically ill patients. Considering the patient's specific condition and potential risks associated with each fluid type, a balanced approach is essential for optimal fluid management.

____

____

____

____

____

____

____

IV Therapy's Influence on Fluid Distribution

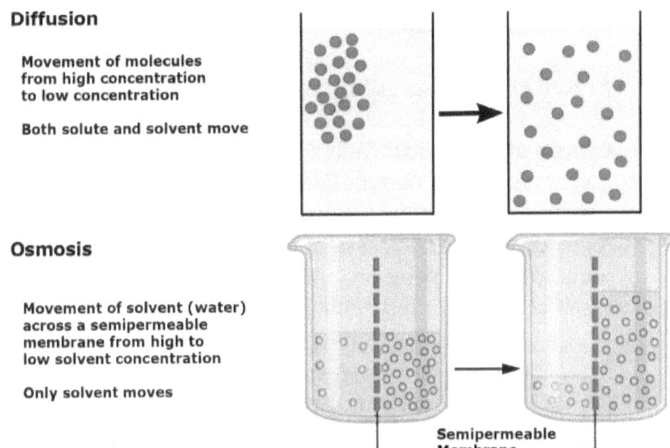

Understanding the principles of diffusion and osmosis is fundamental in medicine and intravenous therapy. Diffusion is the process by which molecules move from an area of higher concentration to a lower concentration. In contrast, osmosis refers explicitly to the movement of water across a semi-permeable membrane from a region of low solute concentration to one of high solute concentration.

Practical Implication: Osmosis explains how the **water** component of IV fluids moves into or out of cells based on the tonicity of the fluid administered. For example, administering a hypotonic solution (lower solute concentration than blood) will cause water to move into cells, potentially leading to cell swelling. Conversely, a hypertonic solution (higher solute concentration than blood) will draw water out of cells, causing them to shrink. Isotonic solutions maintain the status quo, with minimal net movement of water.

Practical Implication: Diffusion is responsible for the movement of **solutes** (e.g., electrolytes like sodium and potassium) in IV fluids as they mix with the blood and distribute throughout the body. This process helps restore or alter the patient's electrolyte balance and osmolarity. For instance, administering an IV solution with a high glucose concentration (a hypertonic solution) will initially increase the blood's osmolarity, causing solutes to diffuse to balance the concentration gradients.

Practical Differences in Patient Care

Choice of IV Fluid: Understanding osmosis and diffusion helps EMTs choose the correct IV fluid based on the patient's condition. For example, isotonic fluids are often used for fluid replacement (e.g., in cases of blood loss), hypotonic fluids for intracellular dehydration, and hypertonic solutions for reducing cerebral edema or resuscitating in hypovolemic shock.

Monitoring Patient Response: EMTs must observe how the patient responds to IV therapy, considering the effects of osmosis and diffusion. For example, administering hypertonic solutions requires careful monitoring for signs of fluid overload or cellular dehydration, while hypotonic solutions require watching for signs of cellular overhydration.

Electrolytes

Sodium (Na+)

Function: Sodium is the most abundant extracellular ion. It plays a critical role in maintaining fluid balance, is essential for nerve impulse transmission, and contributes to muscle contraction and heart function.

Clinical Note: Monitoring sodium levels is crucial, as imbalances can lead to conditions like dehydration, hyponatremia (low sodium), or hypernatremia (high sodium), affecting brain function and fluid balance.

Potassium (K+)

Function: Potassium is the primary intracellular ion. It's vital for normal cell function, including nerve transmission, muscle contraction (especially important for heart muscle function), and fluid balance within cells.

Calcium (Ca2+)

Function: Calcium is essential for bone and teeth health, blood clotting, nerve impulse transmission, muscle contraction, and heart function. It also plays a role in enzyme function and signal transduction within cells.

Clinical Note: Imbalances can lead to tetany (involuntary muscle contraction), changes in cardiac rhythms, and bone density issues.

Magnesium (Mg2+) Function: Magnesium is crucial for over 300 enzyme systems that regulate diverse biochemical reactions in the body, including protein synthesis, muscle and nerve function, blood glucose control, and blood pressure regulation. It also contributes to the structural development of bone and is required for the synthesis of DNA, RNA, and the antioxidant glutathione.

Chloride (Cl-)

Function: Chloride is the most abundant extracellular anion and plays a key role in maintaining osmotic pressure and water balance. It's also important to produce stomach acid (HCl) and maintain acid-base balance.

Clinical Note: Imbalances can occur with fluid loss and can affect pH balance and fluid shifts

Bicarbonate (HCO3-)

Function: Bicarbonate serves as a major buffer in maintaining the body's acid-base balance (pH). It helps neutralize acids in the body, contributing to pH regulation.

Clinical Note: Alterations in bicarbonate levels can indicate or lead to metabolic acidosis or alkalosis, affecting cellular activities and metabolism.

Phosphate (PO_4^{3-})

Function: Phosphate is involved in energy storage and transfer through ATP, helps in bone and teeth formation, and is important in the regulation of biochemical pathways by phosphorylation. It also helps regulate the body's acid-base balance.

Clinical Note: Imbalances can affect bone health, energy levels, and overall metabolic rate.

Check on Learning

What is the most abundant extracellular ion?

a. Magnesium
b. Phosphate
c. Copper
d. Sodium

Sodium ions (Na^+) are the most abundant extracellular ions, which means that among the various types of ions found in the fluids outside of cells, sodium ions are present in the highest concentration. In severe cases, excessive sodium loss (from something as simple as excessive sweating) can lead to hyponatremia, a condition characterized by abnormally low levels of sodium in the blood. Symptoms of hyponatremia can include nausea, headache, confusion, seizures, and in extreme cases, can be life-threatening, resulting in cardiac arrest.

____

____

____

____

____

____

____

____

Why is water the universal solvent?

Water is often referred to as the "**universal solvent**" because it can dissolve more substances than any other liquid. This unique property is due to the molecular structure and the chemical properties of water.

Here's why.

Polar Molecule: Water (H_2O) is a polar molecule, meaning it has a partial positive charge near the hydrogen atoms and a partial negative charge near the oxygen atom. This polarity allows water molecules to attract and surround various ions and molecules.

Hydrogen Bonding: Water molecules can form hydrogen bonds with other polar molecules and ions. These hydrogen bonds are relatively strong compared to other types of intermolecular forces, which allows water to break apart the molecular structures of compounds and dissolve them.

Versatility with Ionic and Polar Compounds: Water can effectively dissolve ionic compounds (like salts) and other polar molecules (such as sugars and alcohols) due to its polarity. The positive part of water molecules attracts the negative ions, and the negative part attracts the positive ions, leading to the dissociation of the ions in the solvent.

Thermal Properties: Water has a high heat capacity and surface tension, contributing to its ability to dissolve substances. It can absorb a significant amount of heat before it gets hot, which helps break down the substances.

Amphoteric Nature: Water can act as both an acid and a base, which allows it to interact with a wide range of substances, further contributing to its solvent capabilities.

The ability of water to dissolve a wide variety of substances has profound implications for both biological systems and industrial applications. In living organisms, it facilitates the transport of nutrients and waste materials. In industrial settings, water's solvent properties are utilized in various processes, from manufacturing to waste treatment.

Fluid Regulation

Autonomically mediated by three systems: Cardiovascular, renal, and nervous. I'll explain.

The regulation of body fluids is a complex process that involves multiple body systems, including the cardiovascular, renal, and nervous systems. These systems work together to maintain homeostasis, ensuring that the body's fluid balance, electrolyte levels, and acid-base balance are kept within narrow limits. Here's how each system contributes to fluid regulation:

Cardiovascular System

Distribution of Fluids: The cardiovascular system, comprising the heart and blood vessels, circulates blood throughout the body. This circulation is crucial for distributing nutrients and removing wastes. It also plays a key role in distributing hormones that regulate fluid balance.

Blood Pressure Regulation: Blood pressure is directly related to the volume of circulating blood and the tone of the blood vessel walls. The cardiovascular system responds to changes in fluid volume; for example, if the volume decreases (such as through dehydration), the heart rate may increase, and blood vessels can constrict to maintain blood pressure and ensure vital organs receive blood.

The intravascular volume varies between individuals, influenced by age, body size, and health status. Gender differences also significantly determine the circulating intravascular volume, with notable differences observed between men and women.

Men typically have a higher total blood volume than women. This difference can be attributed to men's larger average body size and higher lean muscle mass. Muscle tissue is highly vascularized, requiring more blood supply.

Volume Range: The average blood volume in men is approximately 70-75 ml/kg of body weight. For a 70 kg man, this would translate to an estimated blood volume of about 5 to 5.25 liters.

Women generally have a lower total blood volume than men, partly due to smaller body size and lower lean body mass. Additionally, hormonal differences and higher body fat percentage (less vascular than muscle) contribute to lower blood volume.

Volume Range: The average blood volume in women is approximately 65-70 ml/kg of body weight. For a 60 kg woman, this would mean an estimated blood volume of about 3.9 to 4.2 liters.

Influencing Factors

Hormonal Influences: Hormones such as estrogen and progesterone can affect blood volume. For example, blood volume increases during pregnancy to support fetal circulation, reaching up to an additional 1.5 liters by term.

Menstrual Cycle: Women experience fluctuations in blood volume during the menstrual cycle due to hormonal changes, although these changes are relatively small compared to the overall blood volume.
Hydration and Salt Balance: Both men and women can experience variations in intravascular volume based on hydration status and salt intake, which affect fluid retention and blood volume.

Renal System (Urinary System)

Fluid and Electrolyte Balance: The kidneys are the primary organs responsible for regulating fluid balance in the body. They filter the blood, removing excess water, salts, and waste products, which are then excreted as urine. The amount of water reabsorbed into the bloodstream or excreted in urine is precisely controlled by hormones such as antidiuretic hormone (ADH), aldosterone, and atrial natriuretic peptide (ANP), adjusting to the body's hydration needs.

Acid-Base Balance: The kidneys also regulate the acid-base balance by excreting hydrogen ions and reabsorbing bicarbonate from urine. This process is vital for maintaining the pH level of the blood within its normal range.

Nervous System

Regulation of Thirst and Salt Appetite: The hypothalamus, a part of the brain, plays a crucial role in detecting changes in blood osmolality (the concentration of solutes in the blood). When osmolality increases (indicating dehydration), the hypothalamus triggers thirst and releases ADH, encouraging fluid intake and reducing urine output to correct the imbalance.

Sympathetic Nervous System Activation: In response to decreased blood volume or pressure, the sympathetic nervous system (SNS) can induce vasoconstriction, increasing blood pressur, and stimulating the release of renin from the kidneys. Renin is part of the renin-angiotensin-aldosterone system

(RAAS), which increases sodium and water reabsorption, further aiding in restoring fluid balance.

Together, these systems interact finely to regulate fluid and electrolyte balance, ensuring that physiological processes can proceed optimally. Disruptions in this balance can lead to various disorders, highlighting the importance of these regulatory mechanisms.

The Renin-Angiotensin-Aldosterone System (RAAS)

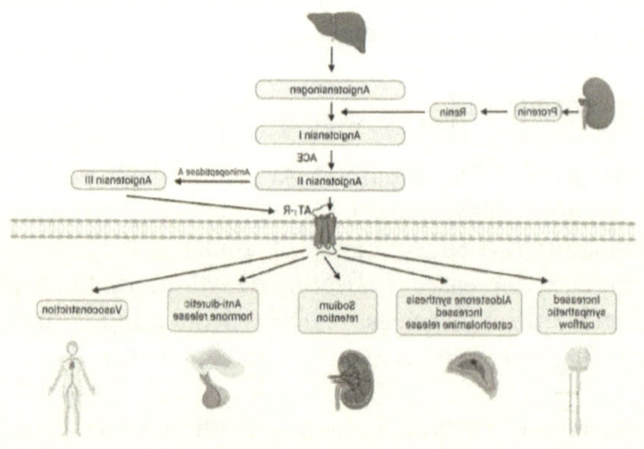

I like to think of this as the thermostat for your body's blood pressure and water balance.

While this looks busy, it can be simplified into a series of basic steps that will aid your understanding of fluid regulation as well as blood pressure regulation. You can directly apply this knowledge to pharmacology when exposed to patients on ACE-Inhibitors.

1. Trigger for Activation

The RAAS cycle kicks into gear when the body senses a drop in blood pressure, blood volume, or sodium levels. This can happen due to bleeding, dehydration, or other causes that threaten to lower the effective circulating volume and, consequently, the blood pressure.

2. Renin Release

In response to low blood pressure/volume, specialized cells in the kidneys called juxtaglomerular (JG) cells release an enzyme called renin into the bloodstream. The kidneys are like the body's smart sensors, constantly monitoring blood pressure and fluid status.

3. Conversion of Angiotensinogen to Angiotensin I

Renin acts on a protein in the blood known as angiotensinogen, which is made by the liver. Renin chops angiotensinogen into a smaller piece called angiotensin I. Think of angiotensinogen as a long train and renin as the signal that causes the train to uncouple, creating a shorter train (angiotensin I).

4. Conversion of Angiotensin I to Angiotensin II
Angiotensin I, on its own, isn't very active. It travels to the lungs where another enzyme, angiotensin-converting enzyme (ACE), transforms it into angiotensin II, a powerful substance. This step is like upgrading a tool to a more powerful version that can do a lot more.

5. Actions of Angiotensin II

Blood Vessel Constriction: Angiotensin II causes blood vessels to narrow (vasoconstriction), which increases blood pressure. It's like squeezing a garden hose to increase the water pressure.

Stimulating Aldosterone Release: It also signals the adrenal glands (sitting on top of your kidneys) to release aldosterone. This hormone tells your kidneys to hold onto salt (sodium) and water.

Stimulating ADH Release: Angiotensin II can also prompt the release of another hormone called antidiuretic hormone (ADH) from the brain, which helps the body retain water.

6. Aldosterone's Role
Aldosterone makes the kidneys reabsorb more sodium and water into the bloodstream while letting potassium be excreted. By retaining more fluid, blood volume and pressure go up. Imagine aldosterone telling the kidneys, "Hold onto that water and salt; we need to pump up the volume!"

7. Restoration of Blood Pressure
Through the actions of angiotensin II and aldosterone, the blood volume and pressure start to rise back to normal. The body closely monitors this process to ensure things don't swing too far in the opposite direction.

8. Feedback Mechanism
Once blood pressure is back to normal, the kidneys reduce the release of renin, slowing the whole RAAS cycle. It's an automated system, like a thermostat, that turns off the heater when the room reaches the set temperature.

Check on learning

Which one of these medications is an ACE-Inhibitor?
a. Propanolol
b. Metopropolol
c. Lisinopril
d. Meperidine

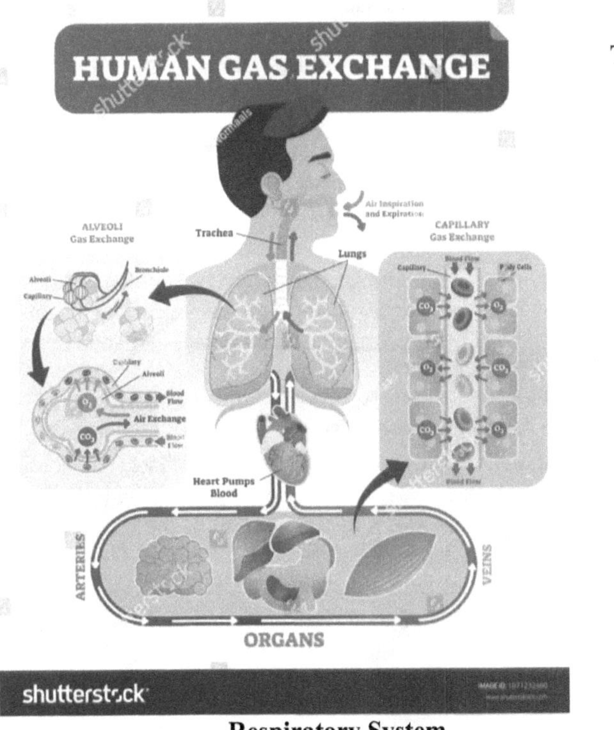

The Respiratory System

Understanding the respiratory system's role in maintaining pH balance and fluid regulation is crucial for an EMT. The body strives to stabilize its internal environment, including maintaining a pH level (acidity and alkalinity) within a narrow range of about 7.35 to 7.45. The respiratory system plays a key role in this process alongside the kidneys.

Let's break it down into simpler terms:

1. The Basics of pH Balance

pH Level: The pH level of your blood is a measure of how acidic or basic (alkaline) it is. The body likes to keep this level just right, not too acidic or basic
Role of CO2: Carbon dioxide (CO2) in the body is closely linked to pH levels. When CO2 levels go up (because of hypoventilation or slow breathing), it combines with water to form carbonic acid, making the blood more acidic. Conversely, when you breathe out CO2 quickly (hyperventilation), you reduce the acidity of your blood

2. Respiratory System's Role

Gas Exchange: In the lungs, oxygen is taken into the body while CO2, a waste product of metabolism, is expelled. This gas exchange is critical for maintaining the right balance of oxygen and CO2 in your blood.
Regulating Blood pH: By adjusting the rate and depth of breathing, the respiratory system can increase or decrease the levels of CO2 in the blood. If the blood becomes too acidic, the respiratory system can compensate by increasing breathing rate to blow off more CO2, reducing acidity. If the blood is too basic (alkalotic), breathing can slow down to retain CO2, increasing acidity and bringing the pH back to normal.

3. Interaction with Other Systems

While the respiratory system adjusts CO2 levels to help balance pH, the kidneys also play a vital role by regulating bicarbonate (a base) and hydrogen ions (acid) in the blood. This renal regulation takes longer than the respiratory adjustments but is crucial for long-term pH balance.
Fluid Regulation: The respiratory system also indirectly affects fluid balance. For instance, rapid breathing can lead to more water vapor leaving the body, impacting hydration status. Conversely, maintaining standard breathing patterns helps to keep fluid loss through respiration at a stable rate.

4. Clinical Relevance

Acid-Base Disorders: Conditions like respiratory acidosis (too much CO2 due to inadequate ventilation) and respiratory alkalosis (too little CO2 due to hyperventilation) are directly linked to the respiratory system's pH regulation. EMTs need to recognize the signs of these conditions and understand their implications for patient care.
Importance of Observation: Monitoring a patient's breathing rate, depth, and pattern can provide critical clues to their acid-base status and help guide appropriate interventions.

5. Practical Application

As an EMT, understanding the signs of altered pH balance, such as rapid, shallow breathing or very slow, deep breathing, is crucial. It's not just about the oxygen; it's also about how the body is trying to correct its pH balance. In emergencies, interventions like providing supplemental oxygen or assisting ventilation can immediately impact oxygen delivery and CO2 removal, helping stabilize the patient's pH level.

Check on Learning

Hydrogen ions play the role of an acid or a base in the body?

Hydrogen ions (H+) are central to the concept of pH, which is a measure of the acidity or alkalinity of a solution. In the body, hydrogen ions play the role of an acid. When hydrogen ions are released into a solution, they increase the solution's acidity. Conversely, when they are removed from a solution, the solution becomes more basic or alkaline. The concentration of hydrogen ions in bodily fluids is tightly regulated since enzyme activity, metabolic processes, and overall cellular function are highly sensitive to even small changes in pH. The body uses various buffer systems, such as the bicarbonate buffer system in the blood, to maintain pH within a narrow range, usually around 7.35 to 7.45, which is slightly alkaline. In the context of the

Brønsted-Lowry definition of acids and bases, an acid is a substance that donates hydrogen ions, and a base is a substance that accepts hydrogen ions. Therefore, in physiological terms, when we talk about hydrogen ions and their role in acidity, we are referring to their function as the defining characteristic of an acid.

Blood Components and Functions

Red Blood Cells (RBCs): These cells are primarily responsible for carrying oxygen from the lungs to the rest of the body and transporting carbon dioxide back to the lungs for exhalation. RBCs contain hemoglobin, a protein that binds to oxygen, giving blood its red color.

Men: 4.35-5.65; Female 3.92-5.13

White Blood Cells (WBCs) are the soldiers of the body's immune system. They defend against infections by attacking bacteria, viruses, and other foreign invaders. WBCs are produced in the bone marrow and are found throughout the body in the blood and lymphatic system.

3.4-9.6

Platelets: These tiny cell fragments are key players in the blood clotting process. When a blood vessel is injured, platelets gather at the site of the damage and stick to the lining of the injured blood vessel, forming a platform on which blood coagulation can occur. They release chemicals that further the clotting process and help to reduce blood loss.

Male: 135,000-317,000; Female: 157,000-371,000

Hemoglobin: Male, 13.2-16.6g/dL Female, 11.6-15g/dL
Hematocrit: Male, 38.3-48.6%; Female 35.5-44.9%

Each hemoglobin molecule
Can carry up to four (4) oxygen molecules
The oxygen-carrying capacity of the blood
100mL of blood = 20.8mL of oxygen with a standard complement of hemoglobin
Loss of hemoglobin impairs O2 transport.
It can occur due to the Oxidation of ferrous iron to ferric form
Methemoglobin Complexing with Carbon monoxide
Carboxyhemoglobin.

The Circulatory Pathway

1. **Heart**: The heart is the pump of the circulatory system. It has four chambers: the right and left atria (upper chambers) and the right and left ventricles (lower chambers). The suitable side pumps deoxygenated blood to the lungs, and the left pumps oxygenated blood to the rest of the body.
2. **Blood Vessels**: These include arteries, veins, and capillaries. Arteries carry blood away from the heart (oxygenated from the left side and deoxygenated from the right side to the lungs). Veins carry blood back to the heart. Capillaries are tiny, thin blood vessels where gas and nutrient exchange occurs with tissues.
3. **Systemic Circulation**: This part of your cardiovascular system carries oxygenated blood away from the heart, delivers it to the body, and then returns deoxygenated blood to the heart.

4. **Pulmonary Circulation**: This is the loop of blood flow from the heart to the lungs and back again. It's where blood picks up oxygen and drops off carbon dioxide.
5. **Coronary Circulation**: Blood circulation in the blood vessels supplying the heart muscle (myocardium):

Arterial Supply:

1. The **right and left coronary arteries** branch from the aorta just above the aortic valve.
2. The **left coronary artery** quickly divides into the **left anterior descending artery (LAD)**, which runs down the front of the heart and supplies the front and bottom of the left ventricle and the front of the septum, and the **circumflex artery**, which supplies blood to the side and back of the left ventricle.
3. The **right coronary artery** supplies the right atrium, right ventricle, and lower portion of the left and right ventricles. It often leads to the **posterior descending artery (PDA)** in individuals with right-dominant circulation, which supplies the bottom portion of the left ventricle and back of the septum.
4. **Venous Drainage**:
5. The **coronary sinus** is the central vein of the heart, which receives blood from the **great cardiac vein**, **middle cardiac vein**, and **small cardiac vein**.
6. Blood from the coronary sinus empties into the right atrium, joining the deoxygenated blood returning from the body.
7. **Capillary Exchange**:
8. Within the myocardium, the arteries branch into smaller arterioles and capillaries, where oxygen and nutrient exchange occurs. After this exchange, the deoxygenated blood and waste products are collected into venules and veins.
9. **Pathway of Blood Flow**:
10. Blood leaves the heart via the aorta.
11. The coronary arteries branch off from the aorta and spread across the surface of the myocardium.

12. Arterial blood passes through capillaries in the myocardium.
13. The coronary veins collect deoxygenated blood.
14. Blood is returned to the right atrium via the coronary sinus.

The path of gas transport via the circulatory system can be described in a circular journey that goes like this:

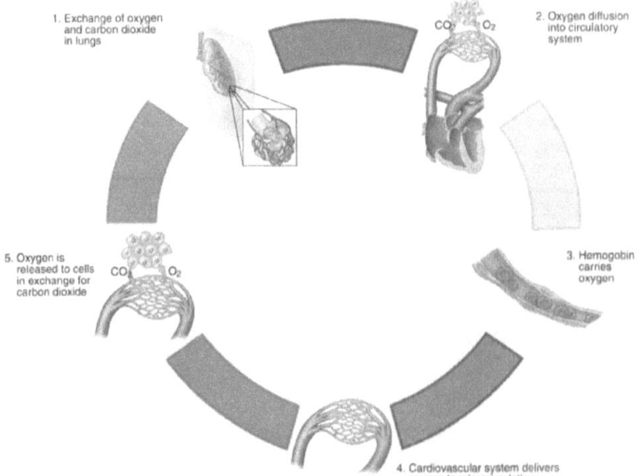

Oxygen Uptake in Lungs:

It all begins in the lungs, where oxygen from inhaled air enters the alveoli, tiny air sacs where gas exchange occurs.

Oxygen passes through the walls of the alveoli and into the surrounding capillaries, which contain deoxygenated blood that has returned from the body.

Oxygenated Blood to the Heart:
The now oxygen-rich blood is carried via the pulmonary veins to the heart's left atrium.

This oxygenated blood is pushed into the left ventricle when the left atrium contracts.

Distribution to the Body:
Oxygenated blood is pumped out through the aorta upon the left ventricle's contraction. This main artery feeds smaller arteries, which branch into smaller arteries and arterioles throughout the body. These arterioles lead to capillaries, where oxygen is released into the body's tissues, and carbon dioxide (CO2) – the waste product of metabolism – is picked up.

Return of Deoxygenated Blood to the Heart:
The deoxygenated blood, now carrying CO2, moves from the capillaries into venules and more prominent veins. The veins converge into the superior and inferior venae cavae, which return blood to the heart's right atrium.

To the Lungs for Gas Exchange:
From the right atrium, blood moves into the right ventricle, which pumps it through the pulmonary arteries to the lungs. In the lungs, CO2 is expelled and exhaled into the alveoli while oxygen is taken up, beginning the cycle anew.

This cycle is continuous, with the circulatory system working in tandem with the respiratory system to ensure that oxygen reaches all body parts and that CO2 is efficiently removed.

Bone's Role in Circulation

Understanding the role of bones in circulation is an important aspect of anatomy and physiology that can enrich an EMT's knowledge base. While bones might not be the first thing that comes to mind when thinking about circulation, they play several crucial roles in supporting and regulating the circulatory system. Here's a breakdown tailored for someone with a working knowledge of A&P:

1. Blood Cell Production (Hematopoiesis)

- **Primary Function**: One of the most critical roles bones play in circulation is through the process of hematopoiesis, which is the production of blood cells. This occurs in the red bone marrow, which is found in the interior of certain bones, such as the sternum, pelvis, and femur.
- **Types of Blood Cells Produced**:
    - **Red Blood Cells (Erythrocytes)**: Carry oxygen from the lungs to the rest of the body and return carbon dioxide back to the lungs for exhalation.
    - **White Blood Cells (Leukocytes)**: Play a key role in the body's immune response, fighting infections and other diseases.
    - **Platelets (Thrombocytes)**: Essential for blood clotting and wound healing.

2. Mineral Storage and Release

- **Calcium and Phosphate**: Bones serve as a reservoir for minerals, especially calcium and phosphate, which are vital for various bodily functions, including vascular contraction and dilation, muscle function, nerve transmission, and intracellular signaling.
- **Regulation of Mineral Concentration**: The skeleton releases these minerals into the bloodstream as needed, helping to maintain mineral balance and pH homeostasis in the body. This regulation is crucial for

the proper functioning of the circulatory system, as calcium plays a key role in heart and muscle contraction, as well as blood clotting.

3. **Support and Protection**
   - **Structural Support**: While not directly involved in circulation, the skeletal system provides structural support for the body, including the thoracic cage that protects the heart and lungs. This indirectly supports the circulatory system by safeguarding vital organs necessary for blood oxygenation and distribution.
   - **Facilitation of Venous Return**: The skeletal-muscle pump mechanism, where muscles contract against the bones, helps to pump blood back to the heart, especially from the lower limbs. This is particularly important in preventing venous pooling and facilitating venous return, a key component in maintaining effective circulation.

4. **Clinical Relevance**
   - **Bone Marrow Disorders**: Understanding the role of bones in blood cell production is essential for EMTs, as disorders affecting the bone marrow, such as leukemia or anemia, can have profound impacts on circulation and the body's ability to transport oxygen and nutrients.
   - **Trauma and Circulation**: In cases of bone fractures, especially those involving large bones like the femur, there can be significant blood loss, highlighting the connection between the skeletal system and circulatory volume management.

5. **Practical Application for EMTs**
   - **Assessment and Care**: EMTs should be aware of the signs of bone marrow disorders and understand the potential circulatory implications of bone injuries. This knowledge aids in the assessment and provision of care, especially in trauma situations or when encountering patients with chronic conditions affecting blood cell production.

Spongy (cancellous) bone is lighter and less dense than compact bone. Spongy bone consists of plates (trabeculae) and bars of bone adjacent to small, irregular cavities that contain red bone marrow. The canaliculi connect to the adjacent cavities, instead of a central haversian canal, to receive their blood supply. The trabeculae may be arranged haphazardly, but they are organized to provide maximum strength, similar to braces used to support a building. The trabeculae of spongy bone follow the lines of stress and can realign if the direction of stress changes.

Compact Bone

Compact bone is composed of closely packed units called osteons or Haversian systems. Each osteon comprises a central canal known as the osteonic or Haversian canal, surrounded by concentric rings, or lamellae, of matrix. Bone cells, known as osteocytes, are situated between the matrix rings in lacunae spaces. These cavities are interconnected by small canaliculi

Compact Bone & Spongy (Cancellous Bone)

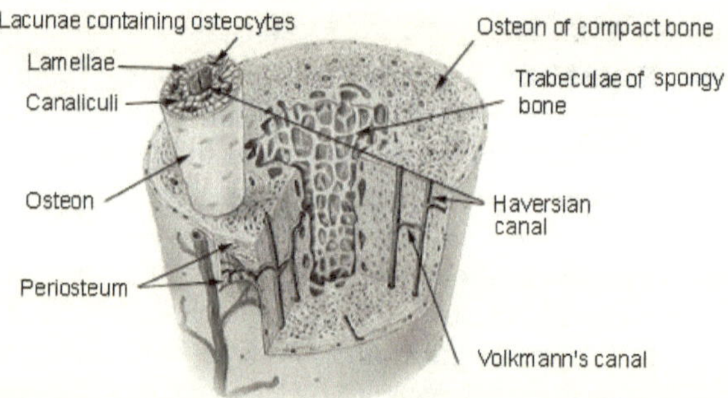

channels that radiate to the osteonic canal, providing passageways through the complex matrix. In compact bone, the Haversian systems are closely packed together, giving the bone a solid appearance. The osteonic canals contain blood vessels that run parallel to the long axis of the bone. These blood vessels are linked by perforating canals to ships on the surface of the bone.

- **Spongy Bone**: Due to its high vascularity and the presence of bone marrow, spongy bone is the preferred site for IO infusions. The rich blood supply in the marrow allows for rapid absorption of fluids, medications, and nutrients directly into the systemic circulation.

- **Compact Bone**: It is less suitable for IO infusions because of its density and lower vascularity. IO infusions require access to the inner, more vascular part of the bone, so sites like the sternum, proximal tibia, and humeral head (where there is a higher concentration of spongy bone) are commonly used.

Blood Clotting

The liver produces most proteins that function as clotting factors and anticoagulants.
The clotting cascade is the body's method of stopping bleeding and involves a series of steps that lead to the formation of a blood clot.
Injury Occurs: When a blood vessel is injured, it exposes specific proteins that are generally not in contact with the blood.

1. Initial Response: The body immediately constricts the blood vessels to reduce blood flow. Platelets (a type of blood cell) also rush to the site and stick to the exposed vessel wall, forming a temporary plug.

2. Clotting Factors Activate: Various proteins in the blood, known as clotting factors, activate in a specific sequence. This is often compared to dominoes falling; one factor activates the next in the "cascade."

3. Thrombin Formation: Activating these factors produces thrombin, a key enzyme that converts fibrinogen (a soluble protein) into fibrin (an insoluble protein).

4. Fibrin Mesh: Fibrin strands weave themselves into a mesh that traps blood cells, forming a stable clot that seals the wound and stops the bleeding.

5. Clot Stabilization and Healing: The clot becomes more stable over time as the vessel heals. Eventually, the body breaks down the clot after the vessel is repaired.

Alcoholics are a patient population that will bleed freely, even from procedures as minor as an IV.

Check on Learning

A common medication that inhibits clotting is?
a. Tylenol

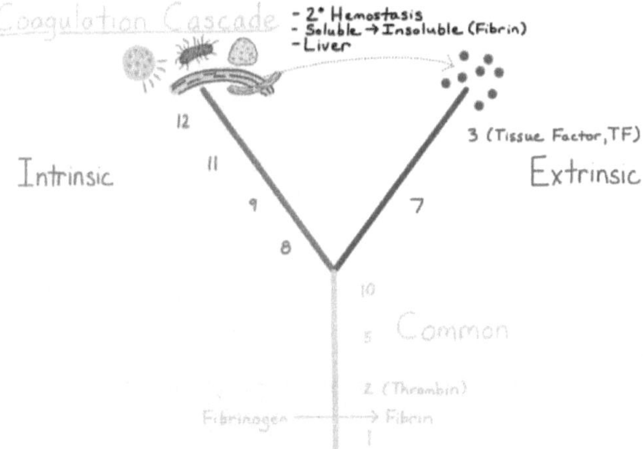

b. Aspirin
c. Fentanyl

d. Albuterol

Aspirin inhibits clotting through its antiplatelet effects, which it accomplishes by interfering with the production of thromboxane A2, a molecule that plays a key role in the activation of platelets. It's important to note that aspirin's effect on platelets is irreversible. This means that once a platelet has been affected by aspirin, it cannot produce thromboxane A2 for the rest of its lifespan, which is about 7 to 10 days. Therefore, the body's capacity to form clots is reduced until new, unaffected platelets are produced.

Alterations in Platelet Function

Platelets are crucial for forming the initial plug at the site of vessel injury. If platelets are dysfunctional or low in number, the body's ability to form a clot is impaired.

Conditions like thrombocytopenia (low platelet count) or platelet function disorders can result in excessive bleeding.

Changes in Clotting Factor Levels:
Clotting factors are proteins in the blood that are essential to the clotting process. Clotting can be delayed or incomplete if there's a deficiency or dysfunction in one or more of these factors. This can be seen in conditions like hemophilia, where certain clotting factors are at low levels or absent.

Medications:
Various medications can affect clotting. Anticoagulants like warfarin or heparin prevent blood clots by interfering with clotting factors.
Antiplatelet drugs like aspirin reduce platelet aggregation and are used to prevent stroke and heart attack.

Genetic Conditions:
Some clotting disorders are inherited. Genetic mutations can lead to either excessive clotting (thrombophilia) or bleeding disorders (like hemophilia).

It's important to know if a patient has a genetic condition that affects clotting, as it can significantly impact how they respond to injury or surgery.

Vascular Access Site Selection and IV Therapy

Identifying Peripheral Vascular Access Sites

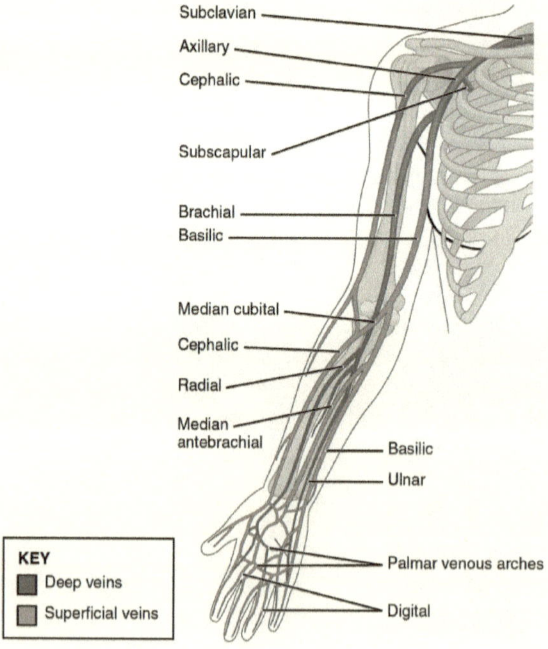

Common sites for peripheral vascular access include:

- **Dorsal hand veins**: Easily accessible but can be more painful and less stable.
- **Wrist veins**: Not typically preferred due to proximity to nerves and tendons.
- **Antecubital fossa veins**: The cephalic and basilic veins are often large and easy to cannulate but can limit patient arm movement.
- **Forearm veins**: Usually well tolerated by patients and less prone to movement.

Advantages, Disadvantages, and Complications of Various Sites

- **Dorsal hand veins**:
    - Advantages: Visibility, accessibility
    - Disadvantages: Increased movement can lead to dislodgement, discomfort
    - Complications: Infiltration, phlebitis
    - **Wrist veins**:
    - Advantages: It may be the only available site for some patients
    - Disadvantages: Risk of nerve damage, patient discomfort
    - Complications: Carpal tunnel syndrome exacerbation
    - **Antecubital fossa veins**:
    - Advantages: Good for rapid fluid administration due to vein size
    - Disadvantages: Can hinder patient mobility, higher risk of accidental removal
    - Complications: Infection, nerve damage, hematoma
    - **Forearm veins**:
    - Advantages: Stable, less painful insertions, suitable for long-term use
    - Disadvantages: It may be challenging to locate some patients
    - Complications: Thrombophlebitis, infiltration
    -

Site Preparation Steps and Factors Affecting Site Selection

1. **Assess Patient**: Evaluate the patient's condition, history of IV drug use, and previous IV sites.
2. **Vein Selection**: Choose a site based on vein condition (visibility, palpability), patient comfort, and anticipated treatment duration.
3. **Site Preparation**:
4. Perform hand hygiene and put on gloves.

5. Apply a tourniquet proximal to the site to engorge the vein.
6. Clean the site with an antiseptic swab in a circular motion.
7. Allow the site to air dry to reduce infection risk and skin irritation.
8. Anchor the vein below the intended puncture site.
9. **Factors Affecting Site Selection**:
10. **Patient Age**: Older patients may have more fragile veins, requiring more careful site selection.
11. **Vein Condition**: Avoid sclerosed or thrombosed veins.
12. **Treatment Type**: More prominent veins may be preferred for rapid fluid resuscitation.
13. **Duration of IV Therapy**: The hand may be sufficient; for longer-term use, a forearm vein may be better.
14. **Patient Activity**: If the patient is active, choose a site less prone to movement.
15. **Medical History**: Consider conditions that might complicate IV therapy, like clotting disorders or infections.

Performing your IV

Check the I.V. Set, Catheter/Needle, and I.V. Bag

Check the I.V. set box and the catheter/needle protective packaging for tears and water marks.
Discard if no longer sterile.
Tear the protective bag and remove the actual I.V. bag.
Check the bag for clarity of fluid and leaks.
Discard if the expiration date has passed, if the inner bag has a leak, or if the fluid is discolored or has sedimentation.
Remove the I.V. set from the box. Discard the set if the tubing is cracked or discolored.
Primary Instructor/Alternate Instructor initiates infusion on volunteers from start to finish, explaining the process and fielding questions as necessary.

PREPARE THE IV

Identify the outlet port and expiration date on the I.V. bag; the spike, drip chamber, clamp, tubing, and adapter on the I.V. set; and the flash chamber, hub, catheter, and needle on the catheter/needle unit.
Remove the I.V. set from its protective bag.
Loosen the clamp (if needed); slip the clamp along the tubing until there is 6 to 8 inches of tubing between the clamp and the drip chamber; then tighten the clamp.

Remove protective covering from the I.V. fluid bag's outlet port without touching the end of the port.
Remove protective cap from spike on infusion set with a twisting motion. Do not touch the end of the spike.
Insert spike into the exposed I.V. outlet port with a twisting motion so the spike breaks the seal in the outlet port. Do not touch the end of the port or spike.
Hang bag on a stand or other object or hold bag up.
Squeeze the drip chamber until the drip chamber is half full of fluid.

Remove air from the tubing of the I.V. set.
Hold the tubing above the bottom of the bag.
Loosen the clamp on the tubing.
Loosen or remove the protective cap over the adapter.
Gradually lower the tubing until the fluid reaches the end of the adapter.
Tighten the clamp fully and replace the protective cap over the adapter.
Protect tubing from becoming contaminated.
Loop tubing over I.V. stand or other object from which bag is hung, if applicable. The bag can also be placed on casualty's chest or under casualty's lower back.
Tear or cut 4 strips (about 4-inches in length) from the roll of tape and hang the strips on the I.V. bag.

SELECT AND PREPARE AN INFUSION SITE

Position the casualty with his palm upward.
Place the constricting band around the casualty's arm 6 to 8 inches above the selected (distal) infusion site.

Stretch the band slightly.
Wrap the band around the arm so one end is longer than the other.
Secure the band by looping the longer end and drawing the shorter end over the loop and under the tubing. This allows the band to be released using only one hand. Be sure the tails point away from the infusion site.

SELECT AND PREPARE AN INFUSION SITE
Tell the casualty, if conscious, to clench and relax his fist several times and then to keep his fist clenched. If unconscious, place the limb below the level of the heart.
Palpate (feel) the vein with your fingertips again.
Open a packet containing a alcohol impregnated cotton pad and remove the pad.
Cleanse the skin at the site with the pad beginning at the site and spiraling outwards.

INITIATE INFUSION
Open the protective packaging of the catheter/needle unit.
Remove the unit from its protective packaging.
Grasp the stem (connected to the needle) with your dominant hand and the protective cap from the catheter/needle with your nondominant hand.
Remove the cap from the catheter/needle unit and discard the protective cap.
Hold the catheter/needle with the bevel of the needle up.

Place the thumb of your nondominant hand about 1 inch below the injection site and over the vein.
Press on the skin to make the skin over the injection site taut.
Position the needle slightly to the side of the vein at approximately a 20 degree to 30 degree angle to the surface of the skin with the bevel up.
Insert the bevel into the skin.
Lower the angle of the needle until it is almost parallel to the skin surface.

Insert the needle into the vein (a slight "give" may be felt) and hold the needle steady.

Look at the flash chamber and check for blood in the flash chamber.

Once blood is seen in the flash chamber, advance the catheter/needle unit about 1/8 of an inch farther to ensure that the catheter itself is in the vein.
Continue to hold the flash chamber with your dominant hand.
Grasp the catheter hub with your other hand and thread the rest of the catheter (not the needle) into the vein (to the hub). **Never reinsert the needle back into the catheter.**
While holding the catheter hub with the nondominant hand, use a finger on that hand to press lightly on the skin over the catheter tip.

Remove the flash chamber and needle from the catheter with your dominant hand and lay the flash chamber and needle to one side.
Tell the casualty to unclench his fist.
Remove the constricting tubing. The constricting band should have been in place for less than two minutes.
Grasp the adapter end of the I.V. tubing with your dominant hand.
Remove the protective cap from the adapter.
Quickly insert the tip of the adapter tightly into the hub of the catheter.

Lift your finger from over the tip of the catheter.
Loosen the clamp on the tubing.
Check the drip chamber to make sure fluid is flowing.
Adjust the clamp so the fluid is flowing fast, but the fluid is seen as individual drops rather than as a steady stream

Check the infusion site for infiltration (fluid leaking into surrounding tissue instead of entering the vein). The infusion site is swollen, red, and cool to the touch. The casualty has greater pain than expected. Clear fluid is leaking from the site.

Question:
What would you do if the infusion site was infiltrated?
Response:

Discontinue the I.V. and start another I.V. using a new needle at a site above the old (infiltrated) site.

SECURE THE I.V

Remove one tape strip from the bag and place diagonally across the catheter hub. Continue to keep the adapter and hub in place.
Remove a second strip and place across the hub forming an "X".
Remove the third strip of tape and place it across the adapter.
The adapter and catheter are now secure.
Make a safety loop with the tubing. Secure the loop with the last piece of tape. The loop helps to prevent the catheter from being dislodged if the tubing is accidentally pulled.
Position the I.V. bag so fluid will flow from the bag, through the drip chamber and tubing, and into the casualty's vein.
If possible, hold the bag up or hang it from a limb or other object that is higher than the casualty's heart. Gravity will cause the fluid to flow.

Tighten the clamp on the tubing to stop the flow of fluid.
Loosen and remove the tape from the loop of I.V. tubing. Start at the ends of tape and loosen toward the middle.
Loosen and remove the strip of tape securing the adapter.
Loosen and remove the two strips of tape securing the catheter hub.

Remove the catheter from the vein by pulling it out at an angle almost parallel to the skin (the same angle used in inserting the needle).
If desired, povidone-iodine antimicrobial ointment can be applied to the puncture site to help to protect the puncture wound from infection.
Cover the puncture site with an adhesive bandage. Covering the site with an adhesive bandage will help to stop bleeding and prevent the puncture wound from becoming contaminated.

Shock

Classically, shock on the battlefield was defined in terms of its physical manifestations and immediate impacts, focusing on the acute physiological response to severe injury, blood loss, or trauma. The concept has evolved significantly over time, but traditionally, shock was often associated with the body's response to catastrophic blood loss (hemorrhagic shock) or severe trauma, leading to a state where the circulatory system fails to deliver enough oxygen and nutrients to the body's tissues and organs, causing cellular dysfunction and potentially leading to organ failure and death.

The classic definition of shock in the battlefield context emphasized the rapid onset of symptoms such as pallor, cold and clammy skin, rapid and weak pulse, shallow and rapid breathing, and a drop in blood pressure. These signs were recognized as indicative of the body's struggle to maintain blood flow to vital organs following severe injury or blood loss.

Historically, the understanding and management of shock on the battlefield were rudimentary by modern standards, with treatments focusing on stopping blood loss, keeping the wounded warm, and trying to maintain circulation through hydration and, when understood, blood transfusion. The experiences and observations of military surgeons and medics in various conflicts have significantly contributed to the evolving understanding of shock, leading to improved emergency medical responses and treatments in both military and civilian contexts.

Categories

(Hypovolemic, Cardiogenic, Distributive, Obstructive, Undifferentiated*)
***Means I don't know**

These four initial categories are broad and generally defined by the event's outcome. Depending on the reference, you may encounter combined definitions or see terms that are not in common usage anymore but maintained for regional/legacy descriptions, such as hypothermic shock, which is retained in some wilderness medicine courses, and hemorrhagic shock, which used to be maintained as a singular category but is generally defined as a type of hypovolemia. (Haseer, et al., 2023)

Undifferentiated refers to a shock diagnosis without a clearly defined or diagnosed underlying etiology.

The Lethal Triad

The "lethal triad" in the context of shock, particularly in trauma patients, refers to the combination of hypothermia, acidosis, and coagulopathy. This triad is a significant predictor of mortality in severely injured patients, as each component can exacerbate the others, leading to a vicious cycle that is difficult to break.

Hypothermia

Hypothermia, defined as a core body temperature less than 35°C (95°F), affects the clotting cascade, leading to coagulopathy. It impairs the enzymatic reactions necessary for blood clotting and reduces the functionality of platelets. In trauma patients, hypothermia can occur due to exposure, loss of body heat through large open wounds, or infusion of cold fluids and blood products.

Acidosis
Acidosis, particularly lactic acidosis, results from inadequate

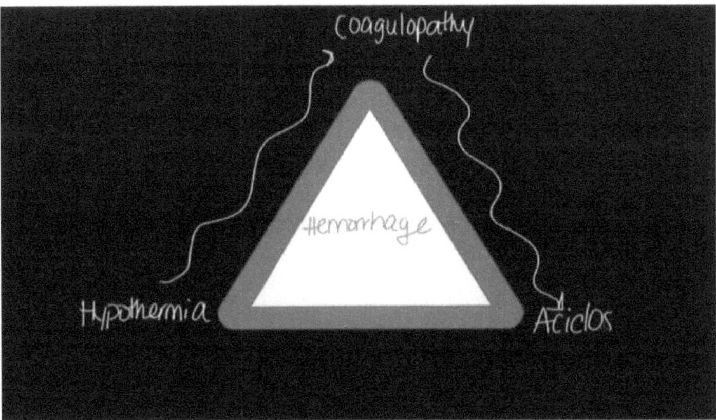

tissue perfusion and oxygenation, leading to anaerobic metabolism. The accumulation of hydrogen ions and lactate lowers the pH of the blood, which can impair the function of various enzymes involved in the clotting process and reduce the efficacy of coagulation factors.

Coagulopathy
Coagulopathy in trauma patients can arise from several mechanisms, including dilution from fluid resuscitation, consumption of clotting factors in ongoing bleeding, and the effects of hypothermia and acidosis. This impaired clotting ability leads to continued bleeding, which can further exacerbate hypothermia and acidosis.

Proposed Expansion to "Lethal Diamond"
Recent literature suggests that hypocalcemia should be considered alongside the traditional lethal triad, proposing an

expansion to the "lethal diamond." Hypocalcemia, often exacerbated by the citrate in blood products used for resuscitation, further impairs coagulation and cardiac function, making the management of trauma patients even more challenging (Ditzel et al., 2019).

Implications

Understanding the lethal triad is crucial for EMTs, as early recognition and intervention can significantly impact patient outcomes. Key strategies include:

- Minimizing exposure to cold and using warming devices when possible.
- Early and aggressive management of bleeding to control hemorrhage and prevent coagulopathy.
- Monitoring and correcting acidosis and hypocalcemia.
- Judicious use of fluid resuscitation to avoid dilutional coagulopathy.

Check on Learning

Hypothermia is defined as a core body temperature less than?
a. 98.6 F
b. 100 F
c. 33 C
d. 35 C

Distributive Shock

Distributive shock, especially its most frequent form, septic shock, results from decreased systemic vascular resistance and altered oxygen extraction. It necessitates rapid intervention to restore adequate perfusion pressure and improve survival chances (Vincent & Leone, 2017).

Evidence and Management Strategies (SEPSIS)

When it comes to sepsis, remember ***IT'S ABOUT TIME***™. Watch for:

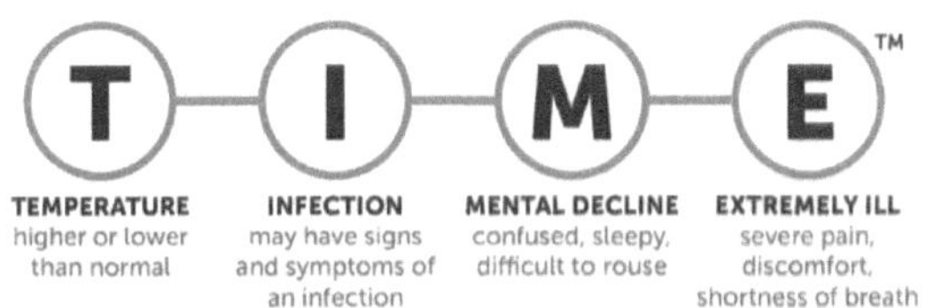

If you experience a combination of these symptoms: seek urgent medical care, call 911, or go to the hospital with an advocate. Ask: **"Could it be sepsis?"**

 sepsis.org

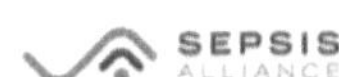

1. **Fluid Resuscitation**: Aggressive fluid resuscitation has traditionally been the cornerstone for treating shock; however, recent findings suggest that a more conservative, physiologically guided approach likely improves patient outcomes, indicating the need for individualized treatment based on the type of shock and patient-specific factors (Marik & Weinmann, 2019).

2. **Vasopressor Therapy**: Managing vasopressor-dependent distributive shock emphasizes the challenge of defining an optimal blood pressure level due to individual patient factors. An initial target mean arterial pressure (MAP) of 65–70 mmHg is recommended for most patients, highlighting the need for a tailored approach to administering vasopressors (Vincent & Leone, 2017).

Systemic Inflammatory Response Syndrome (SIRS) is a clinical condition that results from a vigorous inflammatory response, triggered by either infectious or non-infectious causes. Infectious causes of SIRS may include pathogens such as gram-positive and gram-negative bacteria, fungi, viral infections (e.g. respiratory viruses), parasitic infections (e.g. malaria), and rickettsial infections. Non-infectious causes of SIRS may include, but are not limited to, pancreatitis, burns, fat embolism, air embolism, and amniotic fluid embolism.

Anaphylactic Shock

Anaphylactic shock is a severe hypersensitivity reaction that occurs when the immune system overreacts to a stimulus, typically a foreign substance such as a drug, food, insect sting, or latex. This immediate allergic reaction can cause cardiovascular collapse and respiratory distress due to bronchospasm, which can occur within seconds to minutes after exposure to the allergen. Immunoglobulin E (Ig-E) is responsible for mediating this reaction. Common allergens that can trigger anaphylaxis include antibiotics, NSAIDs, and other medications.

Neurogenic Shock

Neurogenic shock can occur due to spinal cord or brain trauma. This disrupts the autonomic pathway, leading to decreased vascular resistance and changes in vagal tone.

Endocrine Shock

Due to underlying endocrine etiologies such as adrenal failure (Addisonian crisis) and myxedema.

Hypovolemic Shock

Hypovolemic shock is characterized by a reduction in plasma volume, which can severely impair tissue perfusion to critical organs such as the brain and heart. The body's compensatory mechanisms attempt to maintain adequate blood flow to these vital organs, but this can lead to reduced perfusion and oxygen delivery to other important organs, potentially resulting in multiorgan failure (Wang et al., 2013).

Management

1. **Early Identification**: Recognizing the signs and symptoms of hypovolemic shock, such as pallor, tachypnea, reduced level of consciousness, and alterations in vital signs like increased heart rate and decreased blood pressure, is crucial for early intervention (Wang et al., 2013).
2. **Fluid Resuscitation**: The initial management of hypovolemic shock involves appropriate fluid resuscitation. The goal is to restore circulating blood volume, optimize cardiac output, and ensure adequate tissue perfusion and oxygenation (Marik & Weinmann, 2019).
3. **Preventing Hypothermia**: Hypothermia can exacerbate hypovolemic shock, particularly in trauma patients, by contributing to the lethal triad of hypothermia, coagulopathy, and acidosis. Preventing further cooling and initiating warming measures in the prehospital setting are important aspects of managing trauma-induced hypovolemic shock (van Veelen & Brodmann Maeder, 2021).
4. **Comprehensive Approach**: Managing hypovolemic shock requires a comprehensive approach that includes not just fluid resuscitation but also addressing the underlying cause of the shock, monitoring for complications, and preparing for possible advanced interventions upon arrival at the hospital (Zein et al., 2022).

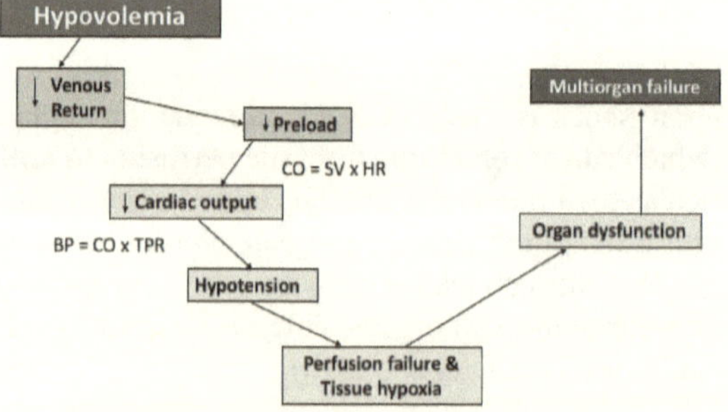

Common causes of non-hemorrhagic hypovolemic shock include:

- GI losses - the setting of vomiting, diarrhea, NG suction, or drains.
- Renal losses - medication-induced diuresis, endocrine disorders such as hypoaldosteronism.
- Skin losses/insensible losses - burns, Stevens-Johnson syndrome, Toxic epidermal necrolysis, heatstroke, pyrexia.
- Third-space loss - in the setting of pancreatitis, cirrhosis, intestinal obstruction, trauma.

Cardiogenic Shock

- It is generally defined as a reduction in cardiac output by 40% or greater. (CO=stroke volume x HR)
- Failure of the heart to pump blood effectively
- Numerous intrinsic causes; left ventricular failure due to MI is the most common
- Numerous extrinsic causes (examples: pericardial tamponade, pneumothorax)
- Manifestations vary depending on the underlying cause

TABLE 9-5 Findings in Cardiogenic Shock

	Left Ventricular Heart Failure	Right Ventricular Heart Failure	Biventricular Heart Failure
Heart rate	Increased	Increased	Increased or decreased
Blood pressure	WNL in the initial stage, then decreases as patient decompensates	WNL in the initial stage, then decreases as patient decompensates	Decreased
Pulse pressure	Narrow	Narrow	Narrow
CVP/right atrial pressure	WNL	Increased	Increased
PCWP	Increased	Decreased	Increased
Cardiac output/cardiac index	Decreased	Decreased	Decreased
SVR	Increased	Increased	Increased
Svo_2	Decreased	Decreased	Decreased
Urinary output	Decreased	Decreased	Decreased
Jugular vein distention	Absent	Present	Present
Heart sounds	S_3	Normal	S_3 or S_4
Edema	Pulmonary	Peripheral	Systemic

Abbreviations: CVP, central venous pressure; PCWP, pulmonary capillary wedge pressure; SVR, systemic vascular resistance; WNL, within normal limits.

Management

- Oxygen Therapy: To improve oxygenation.
- Pharmacologic Therapies: Use of inotropes (e.g., dobutamine) to increase myocardial contractility and vasodilators (e.g., nitroglycerin) to decrease preload and afterload, improving cardiac output.
- Fluid Management: Careful fluid management is crucial; while some patients may benefit from fluids, others may require diuretics to manage pulmonary congestion.

Advanced Therapies:

- Mechanical Support Devices: In cases where pharmacological treatment is not sufficient, mechanical circulatory support devices (e.g., intra-aortic balloon pump (IABP), ventricular assist devices (VADs), or extracorporeal membrane oxygenation (ECMO)) may be necessary.
- Revascularization: In cases of cardiogenic shock due to myocardial infarction, urgent revascularization (percutaneous coronary intervention (PCI) or coronary artery bypass grafting (CABG)) is critical to restore blood flow to the myocardium.

Obstructive Shock

Obstructive shock occurs when a blockage or obstruction in the heart or great vessels prevents the effective circulation of blood. Common causes include:

- **Cardiac Tamponade**: Accumulation of fluid in the pericardium (the sac around the heart) that restricts the heart's movement.

- **Tension Pneumothorax**: A severe form of pneumothorax where air trapped in the pleural space increases pressure, collapsing the lung and shifting mediastinal structures, which can impede venous return to the heart.

- **Pulmonary Embolism (PE)**: A blood clot lodged in the pulmonary artery blocking blood flow from the right ventricle of the heart to the lungs.
- **Aortic Dissection**: A tear in the aorta's inner layer, causing blood to flow between the layers of the blood vessel wall, can lead to a rupture or decreased blood flow to organs.

Pathophysiology
Understanding the A&P behind obstructive shock is crucial for its management. In obstructive shock, the obstruction causes a decrease in the venous return to the heart, leading to decreased cardiac output and inadequate tissue perfusion. This can rapidly progress to cellular dysfunction and organ failure if not promptly corrected.

The Stages of Shock

Shock is a condition that occurs when the body does not receive enough oxygen or is unable to use it properly, leading to cellular and tissue hypoxia. This can be caused by decreased oxygen delivery, increased oxygen consumption, or inadequate oxygen utilization. Shock is a severe and potentially life-threatening condition that can result in circulatory failure. The most common symptom of shock is low blood pressure, with systolic blood pressure less than 90 mm Hg or MAP less than 65 mmHg. **Remember that MAP is a stronger indicator of perfusion than systolic blood pressure.**

A wide range of underlying conditions can cause shock, and there are four broad categories of shock: distributive, hypovolemic, cardiogenic, and obstructive. Each category is caused by different etiologies, contributing to the final shock outcome. Undifferentiated shock is when the shock diagnosis

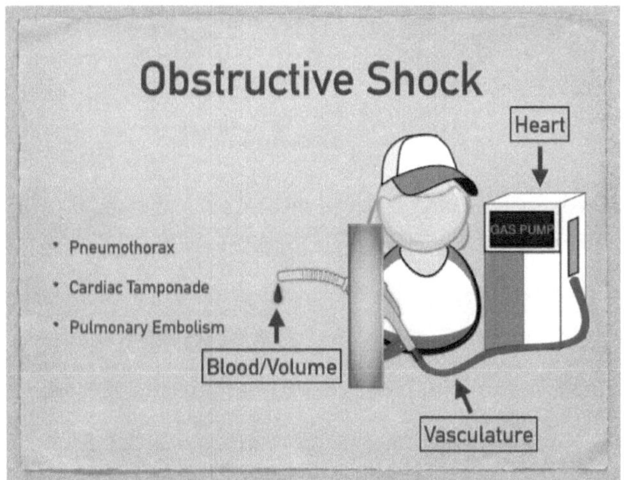

has been made, but the condition's underlying cause is not yet known. Diagnosing and treating the underlying cause of shock is essential to prevent it from becoming fatal.

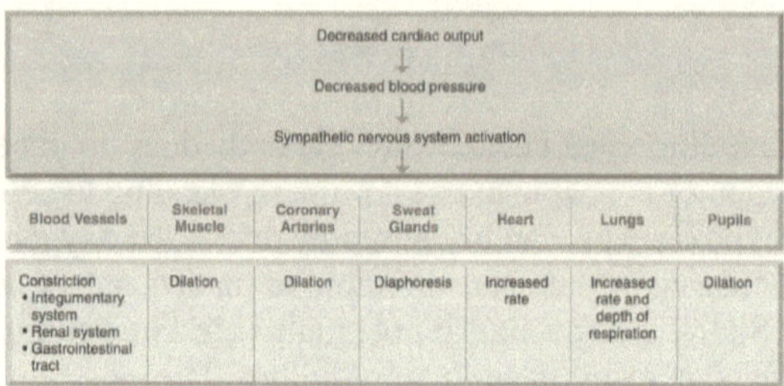

Decreased cardiac output
↓
Decreased blood pressure
↓
Sympathetic nervous system activation
↓

Blood Vessels	Skeletal Muscle	Coronary Arteries	Sweat Glands	Heart	Lungs	Pupils
Constriction • Integumentary system • Renal system • Gastrointestinal tract	Dilation	Dilation	Diaphoresis	Increased rate	Increased rate and depth of respiration	Dilation

The image above describes our physiologic response to shock broken down by body system.

Shock is generally broken down into four stages. Getting ahead of a critical patient's desire to leave this world is incumbent upon the practitioner, recognizing it as soon as they can and then beginning aggressive measures. If your patient is decompensating, you're behind the power curve. Reviewing the four stages of shock we can describe them as follows:

INITIAL
Blood flow to microcirculatory beds decreases.
Hypoxia develops.
Cells cannot maintain homeostasis.

COMPENSATORY
The body uses physiological mechanisms to maintain cellular homeostasis (Increased HR, breathing, shunting of blood, etc.).

DECOMPENSATING
Occurs when the underlying cause is untreated
Life-threatening emergency
Requires early fluid resuscitation and vasopressor support

IRREVERSIBLE
Failure of compensatory mechanisms
Tissues and organs die

Highest mortality rate

When we discuss Multi System Organ Dysfunction

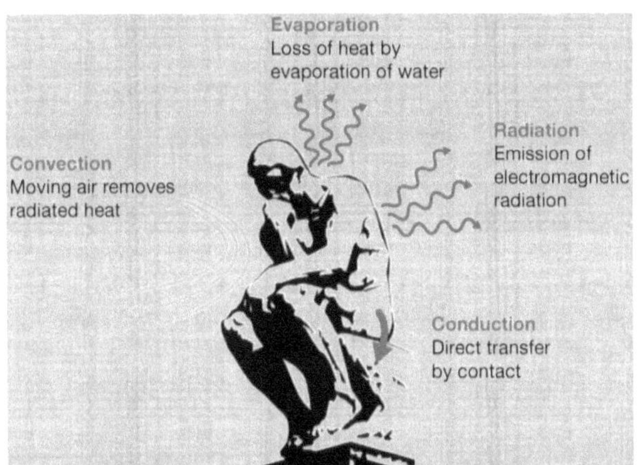

Shock, irrespective of its type, has profound impacts on the body's organs, primarily due to inadequate oxygen and nutrient delivery and the subsequent failure of cellular metabolism. Each type of shock, including cardiogenic, hypovolemic, obstructive, and distributive (septic, anaphylactic, neurogenic), has unique pathways leading to organ dysfunction, yet all result in critical outcomes if not promptly and effectively managed.

Cardiogenic Shock and Organ Dysfunction

Cardiogenic shock, primarily resulting from heart failure, leads to inadequate circulation, affecting multiple organs. Kidney and liver dysfunctions are notably prevalent, increasing mortality rates among affected patients. These conditions require careful monitoring and management, highlighting the importance of recognizing injury and dysfunction early in the management of patients in cardiogenic shock (Lassus, 2020).

Hypovolemic and Obstructive Shock: Pathophysiology and Impact

Both hypovolemic and obstructive shocks result from a decrease in circulatory volume, either through fluid loss or physical obstruction to blood flow. These shocks lead to a cascade of pathophysiological events, including altered maturation and heart failure, or trauma and bleeding causing hypovolemia. Without timely intervention, these shocks can lead to multiple organ failure and death, underscoring the need for rapid diagnosis and treatment (Zein et al., 2022).

When managing our shock patients, keeping heat preserved is crucial. Heat is lost in several ways:

Conduction
The transfer of heat between objects, in contact at different temperatures
Example is a body lying on cold ground (actually touching the colder object)

Convection
Transfer of heat from the body in liquids or gases
Example is wind chill or being submerged in cold water.

Evaporation
Heat loss due to perspiration, on the skin, evaporates and takes heat with it

Radiation
Heat transfer from an object of intense temperature to an object of lower temperature due to the movement of atoms and molecules sending out heat
Example of body heat being lost to the atmosphere or colder objects near the body

Pearls: Shock is just a term. We act to prevent systems from failing.

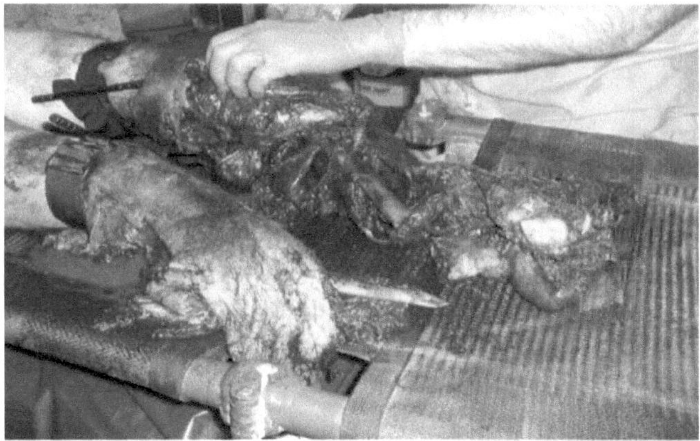

- Shock is a clinical manifestation of circulatory failure and is associated with high morbidity and mortality.
- There are four broad types of shock: distributive, cardiogenic, hypovolemic, and obstructive.
- An accurate diagnosis requires a good understanding of the underlying pathophysiology and clinical, biochemical, and hemodynamic manifestations of the different types of shock.
- Serum lactate level is a valuable risk stratification tool in managing undifferentiated shock.
- Timely diagnosis and initiation of appropriate therapy are of paramount importance as they can prevent progression to reversible shock, multiorgan failure, and death.
- Treatment includes hemodynamic stabilization and correction of the underlying etiology of shock.

Treat the underlying causes (Massive hemorrhage due to trauma, fluid loss due to severe dehydration, fluid shifts due to anaphylaxis).

KEEP THEM WARM. Double-check tourniquets and dressings!

Medical Math

In medical math, two things make your life easier: knowing conversions and knowing how to simplify math problems. A broad range of core competencies comes from having a solid handle on your math skills.

1. **Accuracy in Medication Administration**: The correct dosage of medication is vital to ensure the efficacy of the treatment while minimizing side effects. Understanding how to accurately convert between units (e.g., milligrams to grams or liters to milliliters) is essential to administering the correct dose.
2. **Patient Safety**: Incorrect drug dosages can lead to overdose or underdose, both of which can have serious, potentially life-threatening consequences. Being adept at conversions and simplification helps prevent medication errors and safeguard patient safety.
3. **Efficiency in Emergency Situations**: In emergency care, time is of the essence. The ability to perform conversions and simplify calculations can significantly improve treatment outcomes quickly and accurately. This skill allows EMTs to respond more efficiently in high-pressure situations.
4. **Adapting to Different Measurement Systems**: Medications may be prescribed in different units depending on the context or the country. EMTs must be comfortable converting between the metric system, which is commonly used in medicine, and other systems, like the imperial system, to ensure the correct interpretation of prescriptions and medication orders.
5. **Dosage Calculation**: Understanding the principles of simplification and conversion is fundamental for calculating dosages based on a patient's weight, surface area, or specific medical conditions. This knowledge enables EMTs to tailor the treatment to individual patient needs, which is particularly important in pediatrics and for patients with specific requirements.

6. **Error Checking**: Being skilled in conversions and simplification allows EMTs to double-check their calculations or those of colleagues, providing an additional layer of safety in patient care.
7. **Professional Competence and Confidence**: Mastery of medical math, including conversions and simplification, is a core competency for EMTs. It ensures they can provide high-quality care and builds their confidence in making critical decisions during emergencies.

Given these reasons, proficiency in medical math is not just a theoretical requirement but a practical necessity for EMTs to perform their duties effectively, ensuring they can provide the best possible care to patients in emergencies. No one is saying you can't have a reference card on your person; it's encouraged. Having a basic calculator beyond your phone can be a lifesaver, especially in scenarios where battery life is becoming an issue.

Gram =	Mass	5 cc =	1 tsp	gtts/ml =	Drops per milliliter
Meter =	Length	15 cc =	1 TBS or 3 tsp	gtts/min =	Drops per minute
Liter =	Volume	30 cc =	1 ounce	Conversion	
Gm =	Grams	30 cc =	2 TBS	Convert grams to milligrams: multiply X 1000	
Gtts =	Drops	60 mg =	1 Grain		
Hr =	Hour	1 Gram =	15 Grains	Convert liters to milliliters: multiply X 1000	
IVPB =	Intravenous Piggyback	X =	Multiply	Convert milligrams to grams: divide by 1000	
Mcg =	Micrograms	x =	Unknown answer	Convert milliliters to liters: multiply X 1000	
Min =	Minute	/ =	Per or Each		
Mg =	Milligrams	— =	Divide		
Ml =	Milliliters	- =	Minus	*Don't forget where to place the decimal*	

Converting Pounds to Kilograms
To convert pounds to kilograms, you use the conversion factor that 1 pound is equivalent to 0.453592 kilograms. So, you multiply the number of pounds by 0.453592 to get the equivalent weight in kilograms.

Converting cc/ml to Liters, kg to Grams, mg to Micrograms

1. **Cc/ml to Liters**: Since one cc (cubic centimeter) or 1 ml (milliliter) equals 0.001 liters, you multiply the number of cc/ml by 0.001 to convert to liters.
2. **Kilograms to Grams**: 1 kilogram is equal to 1,000 grams. Multiply the number of kilograms by 1,000 to convert to grams.

3. **Milligrams to Micrograms**: 1 milligram is equal to 1,000 micrograms. Multiply the number of milligrams by 1,000 to convert to micrograms.
4.

Calculating Medication Dosage Using Patient Weight
In an acute patient environment, the medication dosage might be prescribed per kilogram of body weight. If you have a medication order in mg/kg, you will multiply the patient's weight in kilograms by the prescribed dose to get the required total.

Summary of Conversions and Calculations

Here are the formulas summarized for quick reference:

1. **Pounds to Kilograms**: Multiply by 0.453592.
2. **cc/ml to Liters**: Multiply by 0.001.
3. **Kilograms to Grams**: Multiply by 1,000.
4. **Milligrams to Micrograms**: Multiply by 1,000.
5. **Medication Dosage Calculation**: Multiply the patient's weight in kg by the dose in mg/kg.
6. **Drops per Minute**: Multiply the total volume in mL by the drop factor and divide by the time in minutes.

Navigating drug calculations and concentrations involves steps to ensure the correct dosage is administered. EMTs must perform these calculations quickly and accurately, often under pressure. Here are some key points to consider:

Understanding Concentrations

- Medications come in various concentrations. The concentration is usually expressed as weight/volume (e.g., mg/mL).
- An EMT must understand how to read and interpret medication labels and know the concentration of the medication to calculate the correct dose.

Calculating Drug Dosages

- **Dosage Ordered**: Determine the dosage prescribed by medical direction, often based on the patient's weight (e.g., mg/kg).
- **Concentration on Hand**: Identify the concentration of the medication available (e.g., the number of mg in each mL of solution).
- **Patient's Weight**: If necessary, convert the patient's weight from pounds to kilograms.
- **Volume Required**: Calculate the volume required to administer the prescribed dose using the formula:
- Volume required (mL)=Dosage ordered (mg)Concentration on hand (mg/mL)

Administering Medication

- Use the appropriate administration technique based on the medication type (oral, intravenous, intramuscular, subcutaneous, inhalation, etc.).
- For IV administration, calculate the drop rate if necessary.

Calculating Infusion Rates

- Determine the total volume of fluid to be infused.
- Calculate the infusion time as ordered by medical control.
- Calculate the drops per minute (gtt/min) based on the drop factor of the administration set.
- **Double-Check Calculations**
- Always double-check your calculations with a colleague or a drug calculation app approved for medical use.
- Confirm the "five rights" of medication administration: right patient, right drug, correct dose, right route, and right time.
- **Safety Precautions**
- Be aware of potential drug interactions and contraindications.
- Monitor the patient closely for any adverse reactions.

- Document the medication administration, including the drug, dose, route, time, and patient reactions.

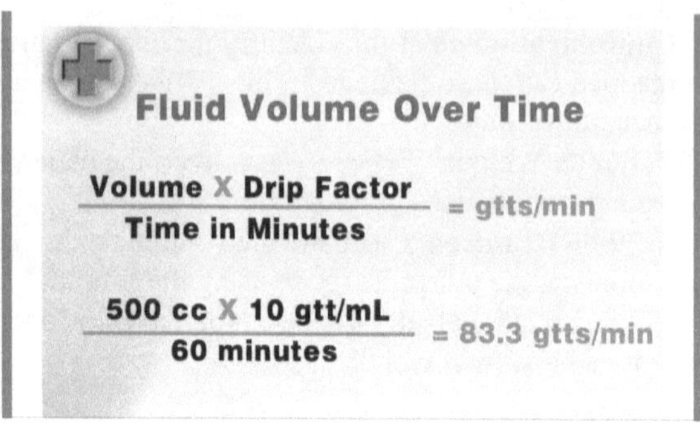

IV DRIP SETS

60 gtts/mL (Micro)
10gtts/mL (Macro)
15gtts/mL (Macro)
20gtts/mL (Macro)

Develop an understanding
There is one (1) 60-minute period in one hour
There are six (6) 10-minute periods in one hour
There are four (4) 15-minute periods in one hour
There are three (3) 20-minute periods in one hour

If infusing 60 ml/hr using a **10 gtts/ml set,** divide 60 by 6 (6 - 10 minute periods) 10 or 10 gtts/min.

If infusing 60 ml/hr using a **60 gtts/ml set, divide 60 by 1 (1 60-minute period),** which is 60 or 60 gtts/min.

If infusing 60 ml/hr using a **15 gtts/ml set, divide 60 by 4 (4 - 15 minute periods),** which is 15 or 15 gtts/min.

If infusing 60 ml/hr using a **20 gtts/ml set, divide 60 by 3 (3 - 20 minute periods),** which is 20 or 20 gtts/min.

All of this is based on the math to reach drips per minute.

Amount to be Infused X Drip Set). = gtt/min
Time in Minutes

Practice Problem 1

Magnesium Sulfate (Understand this isn't in your scope yet but you can still learn about it)

A physician orders Magnesium Sulfate 1g to be administered over 30 minutes for a patient with pre-eclampsia. The Magnesium Sulfate is supplied in a 50mL bag containing 2g of Magnesium Sulfate. The IV tubing being used has a drop factor of 15 gtt/mL. Calculate the drip rate in drops per minute (gtt/min) that should be set for this infusion.

Solution:

1. **Determine the volume of Magnesium Sulfate to be infused**: The physician orders 1g of Magnesium Sulfate, but the bag contains 2g in 50mL. Therefore, we need to administer half of the bag to deliver 1g of Magnesium Sulfate, which is 25mL.

2. **Calculate the infusion time in minutes**: The physician orders the dose to be administered over 30 minutes.
3. **Calculate the drip rate using the drop factor**: The drop factor of the IV tubing is 15 gtt/mL. The formula for calculating the drip rate is:
4. DRIP RATE= VOLUME TO BE INFUSED (mL) x DROP FACTOR (gtt/mL) / Time (Minutes)
5. 25mL x 15gtt/mL / 30min
6. **12.5,** so round up to **13**

Practice Problem 2

D5W Maintenance Infusion

A patient is ordered to receive a 100mL/hr infusion of D5W (5% Dextrose in Water). The IV set available has a drop factor of 10 gtt/mL. Calculate the drip rate in drops per minute (gtt/min) that should be set for this infusion.

____

____

____

____

____

____

Solution

1. **Infusion rate**: 100mL per hour as ordered by the physician.

2. **Drop factor**: 10 drops per milliliter (gtt/mL) for the IV set being used.
3. gtts/min=Volume to be infused (mL)×Drop Factor (gtt/mL)/Time(Minutes)
3. 100mLx10gtts/60min=
4. The drip rate should be set at approximately 16.7 drops per minute (gtt/min) for the infusion of D5W. To make this practical for clinical use, you would round this to the nearest whole number, which is 17 drops per minute.

NOW…!

1. Solving the same problem using simplified math.
2. Go back to the previous problem.
3. Find the mL/min. 100mL/60min=1.67(ish)
4. Multiple by drop factor (10)
5. 16.7!

Practice Problem 3

Amiodarone Drip

Calculate giving 150mg of amiodarone over 10 minutes with a 10gtts dripset

____

____

____

____

____

____

- **Amiodarone dose**: 150mg to be given over 10 minutes.
- **Solution volume**: 100mL (assuming the 150mg is diluted in 100mL of solution).
- **Drop factor**: 10 gtt/mL.
- **Time**: 10 minutes.
-

The drip rate should be set at 100 drops per minute (gtt/min) for the infusion of Amiodarone, given the parameters provided and assuming the 150mg dose is diluted in 100mL of solution with a drip set that has a drop factor of 10 gtt/mL.

Simplified it would look something like this:

Drip rate=100mL×10gtt/mL ÷ 10 minutes

Drip rate=1000 gtt ÷10 minutes

100gtts/min

Vascular Therapy in Adults vs. Children

1. **Vascular Access Difficulty**: In children, especially infants and neonates, veins are smaller, more fragile, and harder to visualize and palpate, making IV access more challenging. This often requires specialized training and techniques, such as using ultrasound guidance or selecting specific sites for cannulation.

2. **Volume and Dosage Calculations**: Children's dosages and the volume of fluids administered are typically calculated based on weight (mg/kg or mL/kg), which requires precise calculation to avoid errors. Adults, in contrast, often receive standard dosages and volumes, with adjustments made for specific conditions or patient sizes.

3. **Rate of Infusion**: Due to the smaller circulating blood volume in children, the rate of infusion must be calculated and monitored to prevent volume overload or too rapid medication administration, which can lead to adverse effects.

4. **Psychological Considerations**: Children may have more anxiety and fear regarding needle sticks and IV therapy. Techniques for reducing distress, such as distraction, the use of topical anesthetics, or child-friendly explanations, are essential aspects of pediatric vascular treatment.

5. **Equipment Size**: The equipment used for IV therapy (e.g., cannulas and needles) is sized differently for children to accommodate their smaller veins. Pediatric patients require smaller gauge needles and IV catheters, which are less invasive and reduce the risk of damaging the veins.

6. **Physiological Differences**: Children have different pharmacokinetics and pharmacodynamics than adults, affecting how drugs are distributed, metabolized, and excreted. These differences necessitate adjustments in drug types, dosages, and infusion rates.

7. **Monitoring and Complications**: Continuous monitoring for complications such as infiltration, phlebitis, or fluid overload is essential in both populations. However, it is particularly critical in children due to their smaller size and limited ability to communicate discomfort or symptoms.

8. **Developmental Considerations**: The approach to vascular therapy in children must also consider developmental stages, as a child's understanding, cooperation, and physical development can significantly impact the choice of vascular access site and the technique used.

The use of a **3-way stopcock** in pediatric IV therapy can have several uses:

1. **Multiple Infusions**: A 3-way stopcock allows for the simultaneous administration of different fluids or medications without the need for multiple intravenous (IV) sites. This can be particularly beneficial in pediatric patients, where vascular access points may be limited due to the smaller size of their veins.

2. **Controlled Administration**: It facilitates precise control over the flow of IV solutions. By turning the stopcock to various positions, healthcare providers can start, stop, or change the direction of flow, which is crucial when dealing with precise dosage requirements for young patients.

3. **IV Management**: The device can switch between an infusion and an IV push medication without the need to

disconnect and reconnect lines, thereby reducing the risk of introducing air into the system or causing infection at the IV site.

Fluid Overload

Fluid overload, also known as volume overload, occurs when the volume of intravenous (IV) fluids administered exceeds the body's capacity to eliminate it, leading to excessive water accumulation in the body. This condition can have serious consequences, especially in vulnerable populations such as children and individuals with compromised cardiac or renal function. Recognizing the signs of fluid overload promptly is crucial for both adults and children, although the specific manifestations and risk factors may differ.

In Adults

Signs and Symptoms:

Weight Gain: Rapid weight gain over a short period is a clear sign of fluid retention.

Edema: Swelling, particularly in the lower extremities, abdomen (ascites), or periorbital area, indicates fluid accumulation.

Dyspnea: Difficulty breathing or shortness of breath, especially when lying flat (orthopnea), can be a sign of pulmonary edema caused by fluid overload.

Crackles in the Lungs: Heard on auscultation, indicating pulmonary edema.

Elevated Blood Pressure: Fluid overload can lead to increased blood volume, raising blood pressure.

Distended Neck Veins: Visible when the patient is at a 45-degree angle, indicating increased central venous pressure.

In Children

Signs and Symptoms:

Rapid Weight Gain: Like adults, an unexpected increase in weight is a key indicator.

Swelling or Puffiness: Edema in children may also be noted in the face, hands, and lower extremities.

Breathing Difficulties: Look for increased work of breathing, nasal flaring, grunting, or a rapid breathing rate.

Oliguria: Reduced urine output despite adequate fluid intake may indicate that the body is retaining excess fluid.

Change in Mental Status: Irritability or lethargy can also be a sign of fluid overload, particularly in younger children who cannot express other symptoms.

Increased Heart Rate: Tachycardia may occur as the body attempts to manage the increased fluid volume.

General Management and Prevention

Careful Monitoring: Regular monitoring of fluid balance (input and output), weight, and vital signs is essential to detect early signs of fluid overload.

Adjust Fluid Administration: It's important to adjust the rate and volume of IV fluids based on the patient's clinical status, underlying conditions, and response to treatment.

Use of Diuretics: In cases of significant fluid overload, diuretics may be prescribed to help the body eliminate the excess fluid.

Patient Education: Educating patients and caregivers about the signs of fluid overload can aid in early detection and management.

Intraosseous Infusions

Intraosseous (IO) infusion is a method of delivering medications and fluids directly into the marrow of a bone, which is a non-collapsible entry point into the systemic venous system. This method is used when traditional intravenous access is not feasible or is difficult to obtain in emergency situations.

Identifying Intraosseous Site Locations

Common IO infusion sites include:

- **Proximal Tibia**: Located just below the knee, the flat surface on the medial side of the tibial tuberosity is a preferred site.
- **Distal Tibia**: Located above the medial malleolus, the ankle bone on the inner side.
- **Proximal Humerus**: Near the shoulder, which is used especially in adults.
- **Distal Femur**: Rarely used but an alternative for pediatric patients.
- **Iliac Crest**: Also an alternative site, typically in adults

Remember that every long-bone is capable of receiving an IO but protocols change from place to place.

Factors Affecting Placement of Intraosseous Needle

The selection of the site can be influenced by several factors:

- **Patient Age:** Certain sites are preferred in children (e.g., proximal tibia) versus adults (e.g., proximal humerus).
- **Accessibility of the Site:** Clothing, injury, or patient body habitus may limit access to certain sites.
- **Previous Attempts:** Previous unsuccessful attempts at one site may necessitate moving to an alternative location.
- **Bone Density:** Conditions that affect bone density, like osteoporosis, may influence the choice of site.

- **Site Complications:** Local site infection, fracture, or previous orthopedic procedures may contraindicate the use of nearby IO sites.

Preparing Patient and Site for Intraosseous Placement

Preparation steps include:

1. **Explanation:** Informing the patient or caregiver about the procedure if the patient's condition allows.
2. **Positioning:** Placing the patient in a position that allows for easy access to the site.
3. **Disinfection:** Thoroughly cleaning the site with antiseptic solution to prevent infection.
4. **Equipment Preparation:** Assembling all necessary equipment, including the IO needle, syringe, and any medications or fluids for infusion.
5. **Pain Management:** Considering the use of local anesthetics or systemic pain relief, especially in conscious patients, as the procedure can be painful.
6. **Puncture:** Using a dedicated IO needle, puncture is made through the skin and into the bone marrow cavity with steady, firm pressure.
7. **Confirmation:** Ascertaining correct needle placement by checking for the ability to infuse fluids with ease and, in some cases, using imaging for verification.
8. **Securement:** Ensuring the IO needle is securely taped and stabilized to prevent dislodgement.

When using the SAM-specific driver, it is important to not let the trigger actuation cause the needle to tilt and change direction or you may bypass your target.

Documentation

IV therapy is important to document, even failed attempts. ESO has a flowchat for IV therapy which is good to use for quality control and helpful for keeping track of individual proficiencies. Your narrative should have a mention of it as well. If you use SOAP as your format it would look something like this:

Subjective:
The patient is a 45-year-old male presenting to the emergency department complaining of acute onset shortness of breath and chest pain that started approximately 2 hours ago. He has a history of hypertension and hyperlipidemia. He states that he has been non-compliant with his medications for the past week. The patient is visibly anxious, rating his chest pain as 7/10, describing it as a pressing sensation radiating to his left arm.

Objective:
Vitals: BP 165/90, HR 110, RR 22, Temp 98.6 F, SpO2 94% on room air.
Physical Exam: Mild pallor, diaphoretic, lung sounds clear bilaterally, heart rhythm tachycardic with no murmurs, rubs, or gallops. Peripheral pulses are intact. The left forearm presents a suitable site for venous cannulation with visible and palpable veins.
Investigations: ECG shows ST elevations in anterior leads. Chest X-ray pending. Blood work including CBC, BMP, coagulation profile, cardiac enzymes ordered and pending.

Assessment:
The patient is likely experiencing an acute myocardial infarction based on symptoms and preliminary ECG findings. Immediate IV access is indicated for administration of emergency medications, potential thrombolytic therapy, and fluid administration if necessary.

Plan:
Administer oxygen 2 liters via nasal cannula to maintain SpO2 above 94%.
Immediate placement of an 18g IV in the patient's left forearm for anticipated aggressive management, which will allow for rapid administration of medications and possible contrast media for diagnostic imaging.
Monitor vitals every 15 minutes and reassess chest pain.

Administer aspirin 325 mg orally and nitroglycerin 0.4 mg sublingually, assess for pain relief.
Prepare for possible anticoagulation therapy post-lab results.
Cardiology consult for further management, including possible angiography.

Avoiding non-standardized terminology in narrative writing

Avoiding non-standardized medical shorthand in narrative writing, particularly in medical records, is crucial for several reasons:

Clarity: Standardized terminology ensures that medical records are clear and easily understood by all healthcare professionals who might read them. Non-standardized shorthand can be misinterpreted, leading to misunderstandings and potential errors in patient care.

Patient Safety: Misinterpretation of shorthand can lead to medication errors, incorrect treatments, or misdiagnoses, all of which can harm patients. Clear, standardized writing reduces these risks.

Legal Documentation: Medical records are legal documents. If a patient's care is called into question, non-standard shorthand may not hold up in legal scrutiny, potentially implicating healthcare professionals in liability issues.

Continuity of Care: Patients often see multiple healthcare providers. Non-standard shorthand can disrupt the continuity of care when transferring a patient's care between providers or departments.

Quality Assurance: Standardized documentation is essential for quality control and assurance processes within healthcare institutions. Non-standard shorthand can complicate audits, reviews, and the evaluation of care quality.

Education and Training: Medical training emphasizes the use of standardized terminology. Deviation from this in practice can lead to confusion and errors, especially among new staff or students.

Interoperability: As healthcare systems increasingly rely on electronic records shared between different systems and institutions, standardized language ensures that records are interoperable and that information is consistent and accurate across different platforms.

Research and Data Analysis: Medical records are often used for research and public health data collection. Non-standard shorthand can make it difficult to extract and analyze data accurately.

Professionalism: Clear, standardized writing reflects professionalism and a commitment to high-quality patient care. It helps maintain patients' trust and colleagues' respect.
For these reasons, it is best practice to avoid non-standardized medical shorthand in narrative writing, opting for clear, concise, and universally understood medical terminology.

Standardized vs. Non-Standardized Terminology

"Pt has c/o CP on adm. Rx w/ NTG, ASA, & BB. F/U in AM w/ PCP."

This shorthand could be interpreted as: "The patient has complaints of chest pain on admission. Treated with nitroglycerin, aspirin, and beta-blockers. Follow up in the morning with primary care physician." It could also be interpreted as utter nonsense even though it's commonplace. This could lead to errors down the road.

"The patient presents with myocardial infarction (MI) and requires immediate percutaneous coronary intervention (PCI)."

This example uses standardized terminology like "myocardial infarction" (MI), which is the medical term for a heart attack, and "percutaneous coronary intervention" (PCI), a non-surgical procedure used to treat narrowing of the coronary arteries of the heart found in coronary artery disease. These terms are universally recognized in the medical community, minimizing the risk of misinterpretation.

Check on Learning:

Which statement is objective an example of standardized terminology?

a. D-stick
b. Amp of sodium bibcarb
c. One 500mL bag of 10% dextrose
d. Doc-in-the-box

Skills & New Drug Education

IM Injection

Selecting the Needle:

- For thin, aqueous solutions, a finer gauge needle (e.g., 25 gauge) can be used.
- For thicker, oil-based solutions, a thicker gauge needle (e.g., 22 gauge) may be necessary.
- The needle length is chosen based on the patient's muscle size and the injection site; adults typically require a 1 to 1.5-inch needle for the deltoid site.
-

Identify Sites for IM Injection:

The most common sites for IM injections include:

1. **Deltoid muscle**: Located in the upper arm, suitable for small volumes (up to 1 mL).
2. **Vastus lateralis muscle**: Located on the side of the thigh, preferred for infants or for larger volumes.
3. **Ventrogluteal site**: Located on the hip, away from the sciatic nerve and major blood vessels, suitable for adults and children over seven months.
4. **Dorsogluteal muscle**: Located in the buttocks; not commonly recommended due to the proximity to the sciatic nerve and significant fat tissue.

Types of Needles:

1. **Gauge**: The thickness of the needle. Common gauges for IM injections range from 22 to 25.
2. **Length**: The needle length can range from 5/8 inch to 1.5 inches. The patient's muscle mass will determine

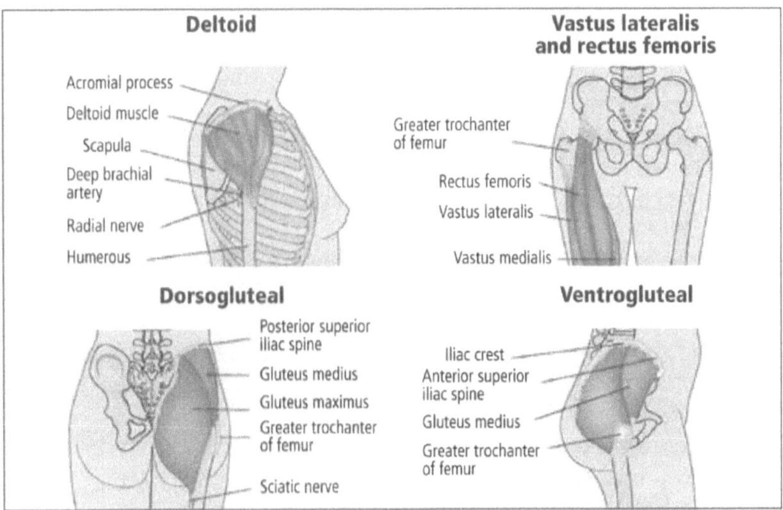

the necessary needle length; more muscle mass requires a longer needle.

3. **Safety Needles**: These needles come with a mechanism to cover the needle after use to prevent needle-stick injuries.
4. **Filter Needles**: Used to draw up medication that may have small particles that need filtering.

Blood Glucose Testing & Dextrose Administration

Glucose is the body's basic fuel and is required for cellular metabolism. A sudden drop in blood sugar level will result in disturbances of normal metabolism, manifested clinically as a decrease in mental status, sweating and tachycardia. Further decreases in blood sugar may result in coma, seizures, and cardiac arrhythmias. Serum glucose is regulated by insulin, which stimulates storage of excess glucose from the blood stream, and glucagon, which mobilizes stored glucose into the blood stream.

Indications for Blood Glucose Testing:
Blood glucose testing is indicated in the following situations:
Monitoring and managing diabetes mellitus.
Evaluating symptoms suggestive of hypo- or hyperglycemia.
During acute illness, where glucose levels may fluctuate.
As part of routine health checks for those with risk factors for diabetes.
Before and after surgery to maintain glucose control.

Appropriate Blood Glucose Levels:
In adults, fasting blood glucose levels are normally between 70 to 99 mg/dL. Postprandial (after eating) levels should be less than 140 mg/dL.
Pediatric glucose levels can vary with age. Infants typically have lower levels than older children, but a normal range is roughly 70 to 100 mg/dL.

Patient Presentations for Glucose Administration:

Signs of hypoglycemia such as confusion, shaking, sweating, irritability, rapid heartbeat, or fainting.
Diabetic patients reporting that they took their insulin but did not eat.
Altered mental status in a known diabetic patient.

Differentiating Hypoglycemia and Hyperglycemia:
Hypoglycemia is characterized by low blood glucose levels (<70 mg/dL), and symptoms often include shaking, sweating, fatigue, hunger, and irritability.
Hyperglycemia is high blood glucose levels (>180 mg/dL) and can cause frequent urination, increased thirst, high levels of glucose in the urine, and in severe cases, diabetic ketoacidosis.

Aspects of Dextrose Administration:
Therapeutic Effects: Increases blood glucose levels.
Indications: Hypoglycemia or suspected hypoglycemia.
Contraindications: Intracranial hemorrhage (if using hypertonic dextrose).
Side Effects: Hyperglycemia, vein irritation, and potential tissue necrosis if extravasation occurs.
Complications: Too rapid administration can lead to hyperglycemia and osmotic diuresis.

Local Protocols for Dextrose Administration:

APEX-SPECIFIC 9090 10% Dextrose Administration For Hypoglycemia (Blood Glucose less than 60 mg/dL)

Dosage and Administration
Adult: 25 gm (250 mL of a 10% solution) IV/IO infusion
Alternative: 25 gm (50 mL of a 50% solution) IV/IO bolus
Pediatric: <50 kg administer 5 mL/kg of 10% solution (maximum of 250 mL)

Considerations for Hyperglycemia (Usually uncontrolled DM1 or 2):
• In general, treat the patient, not the glucose value. Treat shock if present.

• Consider NS bolus for patients with hyperglycemia and no evidence of fluid overload.
• Pediatric patients with concern for DKA should not exceed 10-20 mL/kg of fluids.

Importance of Drawing a Tube of Blood Prior to Dextrose: It's essential for accurately assessing the blood glucose level before intervention and for medical record documentation. Additionally, it can provide a baseline in case of adverse reactions.

Test your glucometer prior to shift assumption with the provided testing fluids

Zofran

Ondansetron, commonly known as Zofran, is a medication used to prevent nausea and vomiting caused by various factors, including chemotherapy, radiation therapy, and surgery.

1. **General Factors Associated with Nausea and Vomiting:**
    - Gastrointestinal disorders (e.g., gastritis, peptic ulcers, gastroparesis).
    - Central causes like migraines, motion sickness, or vertigo.
    - Pregnancy, particularly during the first trimester.
    - Infectious illnesses, such as gastroenteritis.
    - Adverse reactions to medications or anesthesia.
    - Metabolic imbalances, like diabetic ketoacidosis.
    - Psychological factors such as anxiety or stress.
    - Chemotherapy or radiation therapy.

2. **Patient Presentation Requiring Ondansetron:**
    - Patients undergoing chemotherapy or radiation therapy who are experiencing or are expected to experience nausea and vomiting.
    - Postoperative patients who are experiencing nausea and vomiting.
    - Patients with gastroenteritis or other illnesses where nausea and vomiting are significant symptoms and are leading to dehydration or inability to tolerate oral intake.

3. **Aspects of Ondansetron Administration in Adults:**
    - **Therapeutic Effects:** Ondansetron blocks the actions of chemicals in the body that can trigger nausea and vomiting, specifically by antagonizing serotonin receptors.
    - **Indications:** Prevention and treatment of nausea and vomiting associated with chemotherapy, radiation therapy, surgery, and certain gastrointestinal disorders.
    - **Contraindications:** Known hypersensitivity to ondansetron or components of its formulation. Caution should be used in patients with congenital long QT syndrome, those with electrolyte abnormalities, and those on other medications that can prolong the QT interval.
    - **Side Effects:** Headache, constipation, diarrhea, dizziness, and fatigue. Rarely, it can cause serious side effects such as QT prolongation or Serotonin Syndrome when combined with other serotonergic drugs.
    - **Complications with Administration:** If administered too rapidly intravenously, it can cause a transient drop in blood pressure or even rare cardiac arrhythmias due to QT prolongation.

Administration of Ondansetron

**Clinical note about Zofran*

Ondansetron (Zofran) is most effective when used to prevent nausea and vomiting rather than stopping it once it has already started. This is because of several factors:

1. ***Absorption:** If a patient is already vomiting, the ability of their body to absorb oral medications is compromised. Ondansetron taken orally may be vomited before it has a chance to be absorbed into the bloodstream and start working.*
2. ***Pharmacokinetics:** The therapeutic effects of ondansetron involve blocking the action of serotonin at certain receptors (5-HT3 receptors) in the brain and gut. This action is more effective in preventing the activation of the vomiting reflex rather than stopping it once it has started, as by that point, other pathways and receptors may also be involved.*
3. ***Gastrointestinal Motility:** Vomiting can be associated with slowed gastrointestinal motility, which means that even if ondansetron is absorbed, its movement through the gastrointestinal system to its site of action may be delayed.*
4. ***Complexity of Vomiting Reflex:** Nausea and vomiting are controlled by a complex reflex that involves multiple triggers and pathways, including the chemoreceptor trigger zone (CTZ) and the vomiting center in the brain. Once the reflex has been fully triggered, it may be difficult for ondansetron, which primarily blocks serotonin, to fully suppress the reflex because other neurotransmitters such as dopamine and substance P (Neuropeptide) are also involved.*
5. ***Severity of the Underlying Cause:** If the cause of nausea and vomiting is severe, such as with certain chemotherapies or radiation therapies, the stimulus for*

vomiting may be too strong for ondansetron to counteract effectively once vomiting has commenced.

6.

For these reasons, ondansetron and other antiemetics are often administered before chemotherapy or surgery, or at the first sign of nausea, to prevent vomiting from occurring. If vomiting is already underway, alternative treatments, including other classes of antiemetics or different routes of administration (such as intravenous), may be necessary to control the symptoms effectively.

IM Epinephrine

Anaphylactic shock, or anaphylaxis, is a severe, potentially life-threatening allergic reaction that can occur rapidly. Here's an overview of the factors associated with anaphylactic shock and the use of epinephrine 1:1,000 for treatment:

General Factors Associated with Anaphylactic Shock:

Allergens: Common triggers include foods (like peanuts, shellfish), medications (like penicillin), insect stings (bees, wasps), and latex.
Previous Reactions: Prior history of anaphylaxis increases the risk of future episodes.
Atopy: Individuals with atopic diseases such as asthma, eczema, or allergic rhinitis may be more prone to anaphylaxis.
Patient Presentation Requiring Epinephrine 1:1,000:

Sudden onset of skin reactions like hives, flushed or pale skin.
A sense of impending doom, anxiety, or confusion.
Swelling of the face, eyes, lips, throat, and tongue, leading to difficulty swallowing or breathing.
Respiratory symptoms such as wheezing or shortness of breath.
Gastrointestinal symptoms including abdominal pain, vomiting, or diarrhea.
Cardiovascular symptoms like rapid heartbeat, dizziness, fainting, or low blood pressure indicating shock.

Aspects of Epinephrine 1:1,000 Administration:

Therapeutic Effects:
Counteracts the effects of anaphylaxis by decreasing vasodilation, increasing blood pressure, reducing swelling, and relaxing the muscles in the airways.
Indications:
Treatment of anaphylactic reactions in emergency situations.
Contraindications:
There are few absolute contraindications to epinephrine in the context of anaphylaxis, as it is a life-saving medication. However, caution is advised in patients with certain cardiovascular diseases.
Side Effects:
Palpitations, tachycardia, anxiety, headache, tremor, hypertension, and dizziness.
Complications with Administration:
Overdose can cause severe hypertension, ventricular arrhythmias, pulmonary edema, and myocardial infarction.

Situations for Physician Consultation for Albuterol:

If the patient has a history of heart disease or is on other medications that might interact with albuterol.
If there is an insufficient response to initial treatment or if symptoms worsen.
When considering albuterol for young children or pregnant women.
In cases of a severe asthma attack that does not improve after the use of a quick-relief inhaler.

Local Protocols for Epinephrine 1:1,000

Albuterol

Causes of Respiratory Distress:

- Asthma
- Chronic Obstructive Pulmonary Disease (COPD)
- Allergic reactions
- Pulmonary edema

- Pneumonia
- Pulmonary embolism
- Acute bronchitis
- Respiratory infections, like respiratory syncytial virus (RSV) in children
- Foreign body aspiration
- Anaphylaxis
- Heart failure

Signs and Symptoms of Respiratory Distress:

- Increased respiratory rate (tachypnea)
- Use of accessory muscles to breathe
- Wheezing
- Stridor
- Nasal flaring
- Intercostal retractions (the skin sucks in between the ribs during inspiration)
- Cyanosis (bluish discoloration of the skin due to poor oxygenation)
- Altered mental status
- Inability to speak in full sentences
- Tripod positioning
- Gasping for air

Patient Presentation Requiring the Administration of Albuterol:

- Wheezing and/or coughing indicating bronchospasm
- Difficulty breathing with a history of asthma or other obstructive airway diseases
- Signs of an acute asthma exacerbation
- History of chronic respiratory conditions with acute worsening of symptoms

Aspects of Albuterol Administration:

- **Therapeutic Effects:**
    - Bronchodilation (opening of the airways)
    - Relief of bronchospasm
    - Decrease in airway resistance
    - Increased airflow to the lungs

- **Indications:**
    - Asthma exacerbation
    - Reversible obstructive airway disease
    - Bronchospasm in COPD
- **Contraindications:**
    - Hypersensitivity to albuterol or its components
    - Tachyarrhythmia, especially when related to cardiac arrhythmias
- **Side Effects:**
    - Tachycardia
    - Anxiety or nervousness
    - Tremors
    - Headache
    - Palpitations
    - Dizziness
- **Complications with Administration:**
    - Excessive use can lead to worsening oxygenation and potential respiratory failure
    - Overuse can cause tachyphylaxis, where the patient's response to the drug diminishes

Situations for Physician Consultation for the Administration of Albuterol:

- If the patient does not show improvement or worsens after albuterol administration
- Presence of contraindications or potential drug interactions
- When treating patients with significant cardiac history due to the risk of arrhythmia
- Severe respiratory distress where advanced interventions might be necessary
-

Local Protocols for the Administration of Albuterol

Narcan

When discussing the general factors that may cause an alteration in a patient's behavior, several considerations come into play.

Such factors include, but are not limited to, medical conditions (like hypoglycemia or neurological disorders), psychiatric conditions (like schizophrenia or mood disorders), substance abuse, medications, trauma, and infections.

Regarding the patient presentation that may require the administration of Narcan (naloxone), it is typically in the context of opioid overdose. Patients may present with respiratory depression, altered mental status, pinpoint pupils, and potential evidence of opioid use.

Narcan can be administered through various routes, each with its advantages and disadvantages. Intravenous administration acts rapidly and is easily titrable but requires venous access, which may not be readily available. Intranasal administration does not require venous access and is less invasive but may have a slightly slower onset and can be less effective if the patient has nasal obstructions or epistaxis.

The importance of patient and provider safety prior to and after administration of Narcan is crucial. Before administration, it is important to ensure the scene is safe from potential violence or environmental hazards. After administration, providers must be prepared for the patient to become agitated or combative as the reversal of opioid effects can lead to acute withdrawal symptoms.

For Narcan administration in adults and pediatric patients, here are the key aspects to identify:

- Therapeutic effects: Rapid reversal of opioid-induced CNS and respiratory depression.
- Indications: Suspected opioid overdose with signs of respiratory and CNS depression.
- Contraindications: Known hypersensitivity to naloxone. Caution in opioid-dependent patients due to withdrawal risk.
- Side effects: May include agitation, nausea, vomiting, sweating, tachycardia, and withdrawal symptoms in opioid-dependent patients.

- Complications with administration: Precipitation of severe opioid withdrawal, potential for aspiration if vomiting occurs, and potential for acute lung injury.

Check on Learning

IM Epinephrine 1:1000 is given for:

a. Cardiogenic Shock
b. Neurogenic Shock
c. Anaphylactic Shock
d. As a vasopressor

Atrovent

Atrovent, known generically as ipratropium bromide, is a bronchodilator medication commonly used in the management of respiratory conditions such as chronic obstructive pulmonary disease (COPD) and asthma. Its primary action is to relax the muscles around the airways, leading to an opening of the airways and easier breathing for the patient. This medication is particularly beneficial in treating airway constriction and is often administered via an inhaler or a nebulizer for direct effect on the respiratory tract.

Indications

Atrovent is indicated for the management of bronchospasm associated with COPD, including chronic bronchitis and emphysema. It is also used for asthma management, although it may not be the first-line treatment in all cases. The medication works by inhibiting the action of acetylcholine on muscarinic receptors in the airways, leading to bronchodilation and improved airflow.

Contraindications

The use of Atrovent is contraindicated in patients with hypersensitivity to ipratropium bromide or any of its components. It is also contraindicated in individuals who have had allergic reactions to atropine or its derivatives. Care should be taken when prescribing Atrovent to patients with narrow-angle glaucoma, prostate enlargement, or bladder neck obstruction due to the potential for exacerbation of these conditions.

Side Effects

Common side effects associated with Atrovent therapy include dry mouth, constipation, blurred vision, dizziness, headache, and urinary retention. These side effects are typically mild and often decrease with continued medication use. However, patients should be monitored for any adverse effects, especially those with pre-existing conditions that anticholinergic medications could exacerbate. Serious side effects are rare but can include difficulty breathing, swelling of the face, lips, tongue, or throat, and increased heart rate.

Section III

Legals

Expressed Consent

Colorado's Expressed Consent Law requires any driver to consent to a chemical test if a police officer has reasonable grounds to believe the person is driving under the influence or their ability to operate a motor vehicle is impaired because of alcohol, drugs or both.

Legal Fine Print

TITLE 42. VEHICLES AND TRAFFIC
REGULATION OF VEHICLES AND TRAFFIC
ARTICLE 4. REGULATION OF VEHICLES AND TRAFFIC
PART 13. ALCOHOL AND DRUG OFFENSES

Current through the end of the 2004 Second Regular Session of the 64th General Assembly

§ 42-4-1301.1. Expressed consent for the taking of blood, breath, urine, or saliva sample--testing

(1) Any person who drives any motor vehicle upon the streets and highways and elsewhere throughout this state shall be deemed to have expressed such person's consent to the provisions of this section.

(2)(a)(I) Any person who drives any motor vehicle upon the streets and highways and elsewhere throughout this state shall be required to take and complete, and to cooperate in the taking and completing of, any test or tests of such person's breath or blood for the purpose of determining the alcoholic content of the person's blood or breath when so requested and directed by a law enforcement officer having probable cause to believe that the person was driving a motor vehicle in violation of the prohibitions against DUI, DUI per se, DWAI, habitual user, or

UDD. Except as otherwise provided in this section, if a person who is twenty-one years of age or older requests that said test be a blood test, then the test shall be of his or her blood; but, if such person requests that a specimen of his or her blood not be drawn, then a specimen of such person's breath shall be obtained and tested. A person who is under twenty-one years of age shall be entitled to request a blood test unless the alleged violation is UDD, in which case a specimen of such person's breath shall be obtained and tested, except as provided in subparagraph (II) of this paragraph (a).

(II) If a person elects either a blood test or a breath test, such person shall not be permitted to change such election, and, if such person fails to take and complete, and to cooperate in the completing of, the test elected, such failure shall be deemed to be a refusal to submit to testing. If such person is unable to take, or to complete, or to cooperate in the completing of a breath test because of injuries, illness, disease, physical infirmity, or physical incapacity, or if such person is receiving medical treatment at a location at which a breath testing instrument certified by the department of public health and environment is not available, the test shall be of such person's blood.

(III) If a law enforcement officer requests a test under this paragraph (a), the person must cooperate with the request such that the sample of blood or breath can be obtained within two hours of the person's driving.

(b)(I) Any person who drives any motor vehicle upon the streets and highways and elsewhere throughout this state shall be required to submit to and to complete, and to cooperate in the completing of, a test or tests of such person's blood, saliva, and urine for the purpose of determining the drug content within the person's system when so requested and directed by a law enforcement officer having probable cause to believe that the person was driving a motor vehicle in violation of the prohibitions against DUI, DWAI, or habitual user and when it is reasonable to require such testing of blood, saliva, and urine to determine whether such person was under the influence of, or impaired by, one or more drugs, or one or more controlled substances, or a combination of both alcohol and one or more drugs, or a combination of both alcohol and one or more controlled substances.

(II) If a law enforcement officer requests a test under this paragraph (b), the person must cooperate with the request such that the sample of blood, saliva, or urine can be obtained within two hours of the person's driving.
(3) Any person who is required to take and to complete, and to cooperate in the completing of, any test or tests shall cooperate with the person authorized to obtain specimens of such person's blood, breath, saliva, or urine, including the signing of any release or consent forms required by any person, hospital, clinic, or association authorized to obtain such specimens. If such person does not cooperate with the person, hospital, clinic, or association authorized to obtain such specimens, including the signing of any release or consent forms, such noncooperation shall be considered a refusal to submit to testing. No law enforcement officer shall physically restrain any person for the purpose of obtaining a specimen of such person's blood, breath, saliva, or urine for testing except when the officer has probable cause to believe that the person has committed criminally negligent homicide pursuant to section 18-3-105, C.R.S., vehicular homicide pursuant to section 18-3-106(1)(b), C.R.S., assault in the third degree pursuant to section 18-3-204, C.R.S., or vehicular assault pursuant to section 18-3-205(1)(b), C.R.S., and the person is refusing to take or to complete, or to cooperate in the completing of, any test or tests, then, in such event, the law enforcement officer may require a blood test.

(4) Any driver of a commercial motor vehicle requested to submit to a test as provided in paragraph (a) or (b) of subsection (2) of this section shall be warned by the law enforcement officer requesting the test that a refusal to submit to the test shall result in an out-of-service order as defined under section 42-2-402(8) for a period of twenty-four hours and a revocation of the privilege to operate a commercial motor vehicle for one year as provided under section 42-2-126.

(5) The tests shall be administered at the direction of a law

enforcement officer having probable cause to believe that the person had been driving a motor vehicle in violation of section 42-4-1301 and in accordance with rules and regulations prescribed by the department of public health and environment concerning the health of the person being tested and the accuracy of such testing.

(6)(a) No person except a physician, a registered nurse, a paramedic, as certified in part 2 of article 3.5 of title 25, C.R.S., an emergency medical technician, as defined in part 1 of article 3.5 of title 25, C.R.S., or a person whose normal duties include withdrawing blood samples under the supervision of a physician or registered nurse shall be entitled to withdraw blood for the purpose of determining the alcoholic or drug content therein.

(b) No civil liability shall attach to any person authorized to obtain blood, breath, saliva, or urine specimens or to any hospital, clinic, or association in or for which such specimens are obtained as provided in this section as a result of the act of obtaining such specimens from any person submitting thereto if such specimens were obtained according to the rules and regulations prescribed by the department of public health and environment; except that this provision shall not relieve any such person from liability for negligence in the obtaining of any specimen sample.

(7) A preliminary screening test conducted by a law enforcement officer pursuant to section 42-4-1301(6)(i) shall not substitute for or qualify as the test or tests required by subsection (2) of this section.

(8) Any person who is dead or unconscious shall be tested to determine the alcohol or drug content of the person's blood or any drug content within such person's system as provided in this section. If a test cannot be administered to a person who is unconscious, hospitalized, or undergoing medical treatment because the test would endanger the person's life or health, the law enforcement agency shall be allowed to test any blood, urine, or saliva that was obtained and not utilized by a health care provider and shall have access to that portion of the analysis

and results of any tests administered by such provider that shows the alcohol or drug content of the person's blood, urine, or saliva or any drug content within the person's system. Such test results shall not be considered privileged communications, and the provisions of section 13-90-107, C.R.S., relating to the physician-patient privilege shall not apply. Any person who is dead, in addition to the tests prescribed, shall also have the person's blood checked for carbon monoxide content and for the presence of drugs, as prescribed by the department of public health and environment. Such information obtained shall be made a part of the accident report.

Blood Collection

Blood collection tubes are color-coded based on the additives they contain, which are designed for specific types of tests. Here's a list of common collection tubes, their additives, and the tests typically performed with each:

1. **Red Top Tube**:
    - **Additive**: None (plain) or contains a clot activator.
    - **Tests**: Used for serology and immunology tests, including antibody screens, drug levels, and blood typing. When it contains a clot activator, it facilitates clotting and is used for serum-based tests.

2. **Blue Top Tube**:
    - **Additive**: Sodium citrate.
    - **Tests**: Primarily used for coagulation tests, such as Prothrombin Time (PT), Activated Partial Thromboplastin Time (aPTT), and coagulation factors, because sodium citrate acts as an anticoagulant by chelating calcium in the blood.

3. **Green Top Tube**:
    - **Additive**: Heparin (either lithium, sodium, or ammonium heparin).
    - **Tests**: Used for chemistry tests that require plasma or whole blood, such as ammonia, electrolytes, and

arterial blood gases (ABG), because heparin inhibits thrombin and thromboplastin, preventing clot formation.

4. **Yellow Top Tube**:
    - **Additive**: There are two types - one contains ACD (acid citrate dextrose) used for blood bank studies, HLA typing, paternity testing, and DNA studies; another contains SPS (sodium polyanetholesulfonate) for blood culture specimen collections in microbiology.
    - **Tests**: Blood culture tests, cellular studies, DNA analysis, and HLA typing, depending on the additive.

5. **Lavender Top Tube**:
    - **Additive**: EDTA (ethylenediaminetetraacetic acid).
    - **Tests**: Hematology tests, such as Complete Blood Count (CBC), Erythrocyte Sedimentation Rate (ESR), and blood films, because EDTA binds to calcium ions, effectively preventing blood clotting and preserving the shape of cells.

6. **Marbled Top (or Speckled, Gold, or Tiger Top) Tube**:
    - **Additive**: A clot activator and a gel for serum separation.
    - **Tests**: Chemistry tests, such as hormonal assays, lipid profiles, liver function tests, and infectious disease tests. The gel forms a barrier between the serum and blood cells after centrifugation, allowing for easy collection of serum.

Training Skill Sheets

Peripheral Intravenous Therapy

Intramuscular Injection

Intraosseous Needle Placement

Peripheral Intravenous Therapy with Blood Draw

Glucose Testing Diagnostic Interpretation – BloodGlucose

Dextrose Administration – Intravenous

Ondansetron – Intravenous

Ondansetron – Oral Dissolving Tablets

Narcan Administration – Intravenous

Narcan Administration – Atomized

Epinephrine 1:1,000 – Intramuscular injection

Albuterol – Nebulized (optional)

IV Therapy and Medication Administration Skill Sheet
Phlebotomy (Straight Needle Blood Draw)

	Possible Points	Points Awarded
Takes BSI precautions	1	

Explains procedure to patient	1	
Identifies the need for drawing a blood sample	1	
Checks and prepares equipment	1	
Applies tourniquet	1	
Palpates suitable vein	1	
Cleanses site appropriately	1	
Performs venipuncture: (1 pt. each) · Correct insertion angle/direction · Fills blood tubes asindicated · Gently inverts tubes with additivesrepeatedly · Removes tourniquet and needle	4	
Properly dresses puncture site	1	
Manages blood tube properly: (1 pt. each) · Places tubes into small biohazard bag · Labels the bag with patient's name · Secures bag with patient	3	
Documents the procedure	1	
Disposes of needle in proper container	1	

TOTAL	17	

Critical Criteria
Failure to take appropriate body substance precautions
Exhibits improper or dangerous technique
Contaminates equipment or site without correction
Failure to dispose of needle in an appropriate container

IV Therapy and Medication Administration Skill Sheet
Peripheral Intravenous Therapy

	Possible Points	Points Awarded
Takes or verbalizes body substance isolation precautions	1	
Identifies the need for an IV	1	
Identifies the need for blood samples	1	
Explains the procedure(s) to the patient	1	
Checks selected IV fluid for: (1 pt. each) · Proper fluid · Clarity · Expiration date	3	
Selects appropriate catheter	1	

Selects proper administration set	1	
Connects IV tubing to the IV bag	1	
Prepares administration set (fills drip chamber and flushes tubing)	1	
Cuts or tears tape (at any time prior to venipuncture)	1	
Applies tourniquet	1	
Palpates suitable vein	1	
Cleanses site appropriately	1	
Performs venipuncture: (1 pt. each) · Correct insertion angle/direction · Notes or verbalizes flashback · Advances the catheter · Occludes vein proximal to the end of the catheter · Removes stylet and properly disposes of needle	5	
Releases tourniquet	1	
Connects IV tubing and runs for brief period to assure patent line	1	

Examines site for inflammation and/or infiltration	1	
Secures catheter and tubing (tapes securely or applies a transparent dressing, taking care to not block the IV tubing connection.	1	
Adjusts flow rate appropriately	1	
Disposes of biohazards in proper container	1	
Demonstrates correct technique in stopping IV therapy and the removal of IV catheter.	3	
TOTAL	29	

Critical Criteria

Did not take body substance precautions

Contaminates equipment or site without appropriately correcting situation

Exhibits improper or dangerous technique

Failure to successfully establish IV within 3 attempts

Failure to dispose/verbalize disposal of needle in proper container

Peripheral Intravenous Therapy with Blood Draw

	Possible Points	Points Awarded
Takes BSI precautions	1	
Identifies the need for an IV	1	
Identifies the need for blood samples	1	
Explains the procedure(s) to the patient	1	
Checks selected IV fluid for: (1 pt. each) · Proper fluid · Clarity · Expiration date	3	
Selects appropriate catheter	1	
Selects proper administration set	1	
Connects IV tubing to the IV bag	1	
Prepares administration set (fills drip chamber and flushestubing)	1	
Cuts or tears tape (at any time prior tovenipuncture)	1	
Applies tourniquet	1	

Palpates suitable vein	1	
Cleanses site appropriately	1	
Performs venipuncture: (1 pt. each) · Correct angle/direction · Notes or verbalizes flashback · Advances the catheter · Tamponades vein proximal to the end of the catheter · Removes stylet and properly disposes of needle	5	
Performs blood draw: (1 pt. each) · Attaches vacutainer barrel to the IV catheter via Luer-type adapter · Fills blood tubes as indicated · Gently inverts tubes with additives repeatedly · Connects IV tubing to the IV catheter	4	
Releases tourniquet	1	

Attaches IV and runs for brief period to assure patent line	1	
Examines site for inflammation and/or infiltration	1	
Secures catheter and tubing (tapes securely or applies a transparent dressing) taking care to not block the IV tubing connection.	1	

Adjusts flow rate appropriately	1	
Disposes biohazards in proper container	1	
Demonstrates correct technique in stopping IV therapy and the removal of IV catheter.	3	
TOTAL	33	

Critical Criteria

Did not take body substance precautions

Contaminates equipment or site without appropriately correcting situation

Exhibits improper or dangerous technique

Failure to successfully establish IV within 3 attempts

Failure to dispose/verbalize disposal of needle in proper container

Blood Glucose Testing and Diagnostic Interpretation

	Possible Points	Points Awarded
Takes BSI precautions	1	

Identifies indications for obtaining a blood glucose level: (1 pt. each) · Altered level of consciousness · Suspected diabetic · Non-traumatic seizures · Unconscious patient of unknown etiology	4	
Identifies the normal parameters for blood glucose	1	
Checks equipment: (1 pt. each) · Glucometer · Test strip · Lancet or spring-loaded puncture device · Alcohol prep(s)	4	
Explains procedure to patient	1	
Turns on power to machine	1	
Preps fingertip with alcohol prep	1	
Punctures the prepped site with lancet/puncture device, drawing capillary blood	1	
Transfers a blood sample to teststrip	1	
Dresses puncture site	1	

Records reading from monitor and documents is appropriately	1	
Disposes/verbalizes disposal of lancet/puncture device in appropriate container	1	
TOTAL	18	

<u>Critical Criteria</u>

Did not take body substance precautions
Failed to identify 2 or more indications for blood glucose testing
Failed to identify normal blood glucose parameters
Failed to dispose of lancet/ puncture in an appropriate container

Intravenous Dextrose Administration

	Possible Points	Points Awarded
Takes BSI precautions	1	
Completes assessment(s) and determines patient needs medication	1	
Calls medical direction for order or confirms standing order	1	
Lists indications for intravenous dextrose administration: (1 pt. each) · Clinical condition suggests hypoglycemia · Glucometer reading	2	

Checks for known allergies, contraindications, or incompatibilities: (1 pt. each) · Extravasations and tissue necrosis · Requires a pre-administration blood sample to be drawn	2	
Checks medication to determine: (1 pt. each) · Expiration date · Concentration · Correctness · Clarity	4	
Verbalizes the appropriate dosage for the medication	1	
Properly administers medication: (1 pt. each) · Draws up required dosage · Instructs patient about the medication effects · Administers medication in IV port closest to patient-slow push · Periodically flows IV to ensure patency of line · Follows medication with a saline bolus/flush	5	
Verbalizes the need for transport	1	
Verbalizes ongoing assessment including observing patient for desired/ adverse side effects	1	
Verbalizes proper documentation of medication administration	1	

TOTAL	20	

<u>Critical Criteria</u>

Did not take body substance precautions

Did not complete, or verbalize completion of, patient assessment

Contaminates equipment or site without appropriately correcting the situation

Administered, or attempted to administer, a medication to a patient with one or more contraindications for use

Administers improper medication dosage (wrong drug, incorrect amount, or administers the drug incorrectly)

Recaps needle or fails to dispose/verbalize disposal of syringe and other material properly Uses or orders a dangerous or inappropriate intervention

Intravenous Narcan Administration

	Possible Points	Points Awarded
Takes BSI precautions	1	
Completes assessment(s) and determines patient needs medication	1	
Calls medical direction for order or confirms standing order	1	

Lists indications for intravenous Narcan administration: (1 pt. each) · Respiratory depression induced by narcotics · Altered mental status unknown etiology · Non-traumatic seizures unknown etiology	3	
Checks for known allergies, contraindications, or incompatibilities: (1 pt. each) · Hypersensitivity · Narcotic withdrawal	2	
Checks medication to determine: (1 pt. each) · Expiration date · Concentration · Correct medication · Clarity	4	
Verbalizes the appropriate dosage for the medication (Adult and pediatric)	2	
Verbalizes consideration of restraining patient prior to medication administration	1	
Properly administers medication: (1 pt. each) · Draws up required dosage · Instructs patient about the medication effects · Administers medication in IV port closest to patient-slow push ·	5	

Periodically flows IV to ensure patency of line · Follows medication with a saline bolus/flush		
Verbalizes the need for transport	1	
Verbalizes ongoing assessment including observing patient for desired/ adverse side effects	1	
Verbalizes proper documentation of medication administration	1	
TOTAL	21	

Critical Criteria

Did not take body substance precautions

Did not complete, or verbalize completion of, patient assessment

Contaminates equipment or site without appropriately correcting the situation

Administered, or attempted to administer, a medication to a patient with one or more contraindications for use

Administers improper medication dosage (wrong drug, incorrect amount, or administers the drug incorrectly)

Recaps needle or fails to dispose/verbalize disposal of syringe and other material properly Uses or orders a dangerous or inappropriate intervention

Atomized Intranasal Naloxone (Narcan) Administration

	Possible Points	Points Awarded

Takes BSI precautions	1	
Completes assessment(s) and determines patient needs medication	1	
Calls medical direction for order or confirms standing order	1	
Lists indications for intranasal Narcan administration: (1 pt. each) · Respiratory depression induced by narcotics · Altered mental status unknown etiology · Non-traumatic seizures unknown etiology	3	
Checks for known allergies, contraindications, or incompatibilities: (1 pt. each) · Hypersensitivity · Narcotic withdrawal	2	
Checks medication to determine: (1 pt. each) · Expiration date · Concentration · Correct medication · Clarity	4	
Verbalizes the appropriate dosage for the medication (Adult and pediatric)	2	

Verbalizes consideration of restraining patient prior to medication administration	1	
Properly administers medication: (1 pt. each) · Draws up required dosage · Instructs patient about the medication effects · Expels air from the syringe · Assembles mucosal atomization device (MAD) to syringe securely · Briskly compresses the syringe plunger	5	
Verbalizes the need for transport	1	

Verbalizes ongoing assessment including observing patient for desired/ adverse side effects	1	
Voices proper documentation of medication administration	1	
TOTAL	23	

<u>Critical Criteria</u>

Did not take body substance precautions

Did not complete, or verbalize completion of, patient assessment

Contaminates equipment or site without appropriately correcting the situation

Administered, or attempted to administer, a medication to a patient with one or more contraindications for use

Administers improper medication dosage (wrong drug, incorrect amount, or administers the drug incorrectly)
Recaps needle or fails to dispose/verbalize disposal of syringe and other material properly Uses or orders a dangerous or inappropriate intervention

Nebulized Albuterol Administration

	Possible Points	Points Awarded

Takes BSI precautions	1	
Completes assessment(s) and determines patient needs medication	1	
Calls medical direction for order	1	
Lists indications for nebulized albuterol administration · Bronchospasm due to reversible obstructive airway disease (asthma, bronchitis, acute bronchospasm)	2	
Checks for known allergies, contraindications or incompatibilities: (1 pt. each) · Hypersensitivity · Cardiac dysrhythmias associated with tachycardia	2	
Checks medication to determine: (1 pt. each) · Expiration date · Concentration · Correct medication · Clarity	4	
Verbalizes the appropriate dosage for the medication	1	
Properly administers medication: · Instructs patient about the medication effects (1 pt.) · Assembles the nebulizer and connects to oxygen (2 pts.) · Provides appropriate oxygen flow (1 pt.)	5	

· Assists patient with use of the nebulizer (1 pt.)		
Verbalizes the need for transport	1	
Verbalizes ongoing assessment including observing patient for desired/ adverse side effects	1	
Voices proper documentation of medication administration	1	
TOTAL	20	

<u>Critical Criteria</u>
Did not take body substance precautions
Did not complete, or verbalize completion of, patient assessment
Contaminates equipment or site without appropriately correcting the situation
Administered medication without physician order (verbal)
Administered, or attempted to administer, a medication to a patient with one or more contraindications for use
Administers improper medication dosage (wrong drug, incorrect amount, or administers the drug incorrectly)
Uses or orders a dangerous or inappropriate intervention

Intraosseous Infusion – Skill Lab

	Possible Points	Points Awarded

Clearly explains procedure to patient	1	
Selects, checks, and assembles equipment: · IO Solution · Administration set · IO needle and insertion device · Sharps container · Antiseptic swabs, gauze pads, bulky dressing, syringe, etc.	5	
Checks solution for: · Proper solution · Clarity or particulate matter · Expiration date · Protective covers on tail ports	4	
Removes protective cover on drip chamber while maintaining sterility	1	
Removes protective cover on IO bag tail port while maintaining sterility	1	
Inserts IV tubing spike into solution bag tail port until inner seal is punctured while maintaining sterility	1	
Turns IO bag upright	1	
Squeezes drip chamber and fills half-way	1	
Turns on by sliding flow clamp and bleeds line of all air while maintaining sterility	1	

Shuts flow off after assuring that all large air bubbles have been purged	1	
Performs intraosseous puncture		
Tears sufficient tape to secure IO	1	
Opens antiseptic swabs, gauze pads	1	
Takes appropriate anatomical site for IO puncture	1	
Identifies appropriate anatomical site for IO puncture		
Cleanses site, starting from the center and moving outward in a circular motion	1	
Prepares IO needle and insertion device while maintaining sterility	1	
Stabilizes the site in a safe matter (if using the tibia, does not hold the leg in palm of hand and perform IO puncture directly above hand)	1	
· Accepts evaluation and criticism professionally Inserts needle at proper angle and direction (away from joint, epiphyseal plate, · Shows willingness to learn etc.)	1	

Interacts with simulated patient and other personnel in professional manner

Recognizes that needle has entered intramedullary canal (feels "pop" or notices less resistance)	1	
Removes stylet and immediately disposes in proper container	1	
Attaches administration set to IO needle	1	
Slowly injects solution while observing for signs of infiltration or aspirates to verify proper needle placement	1	
Adjusts flow rate as appropriate	1	
Secures needle and supports with bulky dressing	1	
Assesses patient for therapeutic response or signs or untoward reactions	1	
TOTAL	31	

Critical Criteria

Failure to take or verbalize appropriate PPE precautions

Failure to dispose of blood-contaminated sharps immediately at the point of use

Contaminates equipment or site without appropriately correcting the situation

Performs any improper technique resulting in the potential for air embolism

Failure to assure correct needle placement

Performs IO puncture in an unacceptable or unsafe manner (improper site, incorrect needle angle, holds leg in palm and performs IO puncture directly above hand, etc.)

Failure to manage the patient as a competent EMT

Exhibits unacceptable affect with patient or other personnel

Intramuscular Medication Administration

	Possible Points	Points Awarded
Asks patient for known allergies	1	
Clearly explains procedure to patient	1	
Selects, checks, and assembles equipment: · Medication · Appropriate syringe and needle(s) · Sharps container · Alcohol swabs · Adhesive bandage or sterile gauze dressing and tape	5	
Selects correct medication by identifying: · Right patient · Right medication · Right dosage/concentration · Right time · Right route	5	
Checks medication for: · Clarity · Expiration date	2	
Assembles syringe and needle	1	

Draws appropriate amount of medication into syringe and dispels air while maintaining sterility	4	
Reconfirms medication with partner	1	
Takes or verbalizes appropriate PPE precautions	1	
Identifies and cleanses appropriate injection site	1	
Pinches/stretches skin, warns patient and inserts needle at proper angle while maintaining sterility	1	
Aspirates syringe while observing for blood return before injecting IM medication	1	
Administers correct dose at proper push rate	1	
Removes needle and disposes/verbalizes proper disposal of syringe and needle in proper container	1	
Applies direct pressure to site	1	
Covers puncture site	1	

Verbalizes need to observe patient for desired effect and adverse side effects	1	
TOTAL	26	

Critical Criteria

Failure to take or verbalize appropriate PPE precautions
Failure to identify acceptable injection site
Contaminates equipment or site without appropriately correcting the situation
Failure to adequate dispel air resulting in the potential for air embolism
Failure to aspirate for blood prior to injecting IM medication
Injects improper medication or dosage (wrong medication, incorrect amount, or administers at an inappropriate rate)
Recaps needle or fails to dispose/verbalize disposal of syringe and needle in proper container
Failure to observe the patient for desired effect and adverse side effects after administering medication
Failure to manage the patient as a competent EMT
Exhibits unacceptable affect with patient or other personnel

References

Occupational Safety and Health Administration. (2009). Best practices for the development, delivery, and evaluation of Susan Harwood training grants. U.S. Department of Labor. Retrieved from https://www.osha.gov

Centers for Disease Control and Prevention. (2024). Transmission through contact with blood or body fluids. Retrieved from https://www.cdc.gov

Occupational Safety and Health Administration. (2009). Best practices for non-health care employers with on-site health care services. Retrieved from https://www.osha.gov

Occupational Safety and Health Administration. (2009). Amputations: Safeguarding equipment and protecting employees from amputations. Retrieved from https://www.osha.gov

Kohan, D. E., Rossi, N. F., Inscho, E. W., & Pollock, D. M. (2011). Regulation of blood pressure and salt homeostasis by endothelin. *Physiological Reviews*, 91(1), 1-77. https://doi.org/10.1152/physrev.00060.2009

Klein, I. H., Ligtenberg, G., Oey, P. L., Koomans, H. A., & Blankestijn, P. J. (2003). Enalapril and losartan reduce sympathetic hyperactivity in patients with chronic renal failure. *Journal of the American Society of Nephrology*, 14(2), 425-430. https://doi.org/10.1097/01.ASN.0000039673.32489.B7

Navar, L. G., Harrison-Bernard, L. M., Nishiyama, A., & Kobori, H. (2002). Regulation of intrarenal angiotensin II in hypertension. *Hypertension*, 39(2), 316-322. https://doi.org/10.1161/hy0202.104651

DiBona, G. F., & Esler, M. (2010). Translational medicine: The antihypertensive effect of renal denervation. *American Journal of Physiology-Regulatory, Integrative and Comparative Physiology*, 298(2), R245-R253. https://doi.org/10.1152/ajpregu.00624.2009

Esler, M. D., Krum, H., Sobotka, P. A., Schlaich, M. P., Schmieder, R. E., & Böhm, M. (2010). Renal sympathetic denervation in patients with treatment-resistant hypertension (The Symplicity HTN-2 Trial): A randomised controlled trial. *The Lancet*, 376(9756), 1903-1909. https://doi.org/10.1016/S0140-6736(10)62039-9

O'Connor, P. M., & Cowley, A. W. Jr. (2010). Modulation of pressure-natriuresis by renal medullary reactive oxygen species and nitric oxide. *Current Hypertension Reports*, 12(2), 86-92. https://doi.org/10.1007/s11906-010-0095-4

Kassab, S., Kato, T., Wilkins, F. C., Ferguson, R. K., & Cowley, A. W. (1995). Renal denervation attenuates the sodium retention and hypertension associated with obesity. *Hypertension*, 25(4), 893-897. https://doi.org/10.1161/01.HYP.25.4.893

Prasad, V. S., Palaniswamy, C., & Frishman, W. H. (2009). Endothelin as a clinical target in the treatment of systemic hypertension. *Cardiology in Review*, 17(4), 181-191. https://doi.org/10.1097/CRD.0b013e3181a72e8e

SAM Medical. (n.d.). SAM IO Driver. Retrieved from https://www.sammedical.com

www.ingramcontent.com/pod-product-compliance
Lightning Source LLC
Chambersburg PA
CBHW051305250726
48656CB00004B/1480
9798329076691